# Whispers and Moans

# WHISPERS AND MOANS

## INTERVIEWS WITH THE MEN AND WOMEN OF HONG KONG'S SEX INDUSTRY

*Yeeshan Yang*

BLACKSMITH BOOKS

*Whispers and Moans*

ISBN 978-962-86732-8-5

Published by Blacksmith Books
5th Floor, 24 Hollywood Road, Central, Hong Kong
*www.blacksmithbooks.com*

Edited by Stephen Maurice Kettle

Cover design and photography by Tim McConville
www.timmcconville.com

# Contents

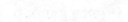

# I

# A ROSE BY ANY OTHER NAME

"What's in a name? That which we call a rose by any other word would smell as sweet."

*– Romeo and Juliet (II, ii, 1-2), William Shakespeare*

A group of apparently wealthy, well-dressed housewives with slightly too much make-up, and slightly too much jewellery, burst into a European-style furniture store in Causeway Bay, Hong Kong. They tore up the bedsheets, knocked over the tables and chairs, yelled, and generally caused mayhem. Miss Fu, the store manager, told Elaine and Wendy, two other assistants, and me, then only 18 years old, to try to reason with the women while she called for the police.

"How dare you stand there so brazenly, after seducing our husbands?" shouted one of the women.

"You chickens [Hong Kong slang for prostitutes], show us what you have that's so good! You don't just sell beds, you whores hop onto them with our husbands!"

Elaine, Wendy and I were scared and nervous. So was Miss Fu, but she stood her ground, hands on hips, feet firmly planted, and responded: "Look at yourselves, you stupid, spoilt bitches! No wonder your men run after other women. Your husbands aren't here. Go and look for them in a whore house!"

The most slightly built of the women was sure this defence confirmed that Miss Fu really did have something to hide. She grabbed Miss Fu's hair and yelled, "You slut, selling beds has turned you into one yourself! How can you even think of being my husband's mistress? Why don't you take a look at yourself? You ugly, dried-up old spinster!"

Ironically, another commented: "Your husband must have poor taste. How else could he fuck a bitch like her?"

The slightly-built one let Miss Fu go and asked, "If it's not you, then who is it?" They looked at us accusingly. Eventually, all eyes landed on Elaine.

"This slut has a mole as big as a broad bean," one of the women said. "She may not be a whore, but she could be their pimp." This stunned poor Elaine, whose jaw dropped visibly. Then, fingers stabbed at Wendy's face. "Men wouldn't touch her poxy face, but they'd love to feel her huge tits." Wendy flushed profusely.

Suddenly, the largest of the marauding women shouted directly at me, "Look at her, thin eyes and thick lips, a born chicken." I was nervous, confused, and angry.

The police arrived within twenty minutes and took the worst of the troublemakers away. There was little sympathy for the remaining women who were left licking their wounds. It seemed to them they were the victims. They were surrounded by a damned pimp, a deserted spinster, whores, a born chicken with narrow eyes and full lips, and a girl with bad skin and annoyingly full breasts; and to add insult to injury, the police were on their side.

For weeks after the showdown, Elaine remained embarrassed at the public ridicule of her mole, and resigned. Wendy reacted badly when Miss Fu continued to remind her of the comments on her skin and breasts, implying blame of some sort. Finally, Wendy sought satisfaction in a settlement arranged by the labour union.

My own supposed "chicken look" was destined to make me the butt of continued jibes. After a row with staff members who were making fun of me, I was fired by Miss Fu.

I was only 18, and found the accusation of having a "chicken look" much more shameful than anything else I could imagine. Years later, I still feel the shame. Even now, as an adult I will look at myself in the mirror to try to see if the accusation has any validity, and to find any sign that I am a good woman.

One of the housewives eventually admitted they had made a mistake and should have gone into the shop next door. The housewives' collective jealousy had erroneously affected the lives of innocent individuals and left me with a powerful memory.

Although confused at the time, with the benefit of hindsight I can see many implications and emotions in the events at the furniture store. The loathing married women have for prostitutes; fear of ageing and loss of attractiveness; competition between females for the same source of security. Objectively, it is easier to blame the most remote party, i.e. the supposed prostitute, rather than the man. Push the man too far and he takes his patronage elsewhere, which creates a self-fulfilling accusation, whether or not a prostitute is the cause.

Imagine if the definition of prostitution was broadened to cover not just cash but security, housing, clothes, and a generally more comfortable life in return for such benefits as companionship, sexual availability, a housekeeper, birth mother, and child minder. It could then be argued that the angry women were simply single-client prostitutes trying to frighten off freelance prostitutes competing for the same source of benefits and security.


Prostitution is often called the oldest profession. It is probably more accurate to call it the oldest business. Despite its many forms, the common factor is an exchange of usually, but not always, money, given in return for sex of some kind. In this context, 'sex' is used to describe any benefit arriving from a person of the opposite sex: non-contact companionship, friendly affection, outings as an apparent couple, all the way through to full sexual intercourse and its many variations.

Whenever and whatever the demand, there has always been a supply, and vice versa. Which drives which? Chickens and eggs in an eternal circle.

In literature and the visual arts, the prostitute is typically portrayed by reference to quite clearly defined clichés: a superficially sweet and appealing creature hiding an underlying, hard-edged cynicism; a downtrodden, used and abused wretch; or a happy hooker in full control acting out of choice, living proof of Darwin's notion that the female chooses the male. This was a shocking concept to Darwin's male contemporaries, and despite its compatibility with biological evolution, it remains uncomfortably at odds with much feminist thinking on the subject of *female* sex workers. The feminist view of *male* sex workers is rather more fuzzy.

Prostitution is a classic case of proximity determining perception. In another country, it may be seen as a fascinating aspect of an exotic culture, something different and exciting. In the next town, it is a social ill, about which something really should be done. In the street in which one lives, it is a terrible, disgusting, immoral, depraved business operated by cheap criminals and even cheaper women.

In truth, people who suppose themselves to be morally superior would rather not acknowledge the existence of prostitution in their own society, its existence being a reflection of aspects of self. Such prejudice is deeply rooted. It serves to reinforce notions of moral superiority and justifies a lack of concern about the welfare and dignity of prostitutes.

Pragmatically, however uncomfortable it may be, societies ought to accept that prostitution is here to stay. If all the might of the United States could not eradicate the urge to drink alcoholic beverages during the Prohibition era, then eradicating an aspect of hormonally driven human behaviour, fundamental to existence, is not an initiative likely to succeed.

In Hong Kong today, it is possible to find those involved in 'public relations', massage girls, karaoke hostesses, house hookers and streetwalkers without too much difficulty.

*Police Crackdown on Prostitution* and *Women's Prison Cells Jammed* are common themes in Hong Kong newspaper headlines. Political parties, hand-in-hand with local community representatives, take to the streets to demonstrate against prostitution in peaceful neighbourhoods. Voluntary groups who care for the prostitutes protest that political parties use an anti-prostitution stance to gain political capital. Counter demonstrations, although attracting small numbers wearing masks, provide an interesting if not overwhelming spectacle, holding banners stating "Prostitute Rights = Human Rights".

Should prostitution be legalised? Should red-light districts be set up? What impact does prostitution have on youngsters? What effect does it have on community and family life? These controversial questions frequently initiate heated debates among women's groups, religious organisations, feminists, political parties, neighbourhood communities and various government agencies.

A British Catholic nun once told me an interesting story. During the course of doing social work, her co-worker once helped a pretty girl who was a college graduate working as a prostitute in a nightclub. The young girl spent her hard-earned money on young male prostitutes. My curiosity was aroused by this seeming paradox, and I was interested to find other examples of apparently contradictory behaviour.

Idly surfing the internet one day, I found the website of Norma Jean Almodovar, an established, successful police officer who, at the age of 32, decided to leave the Los Angeles Police Department and sell her body. She wrote a short article entitled 'Sex/Prostitution/Power', in which she claimed that prostitution out of choice is not pitiful at all, but empowers women to enjoy sex without the emotional burdens associated with steady relationships. Taking an agreed service fee from a man freed her from the need to submit to a partner, a husband or a boss, as 'respectable' women do. In fact, she encourages all women to consider prostitution as a profession.

Are these examples of the mythical 'happy hooker'? Despite my curiosity and best efforts, I could not find the co-worker of the British nun to verify her story.

We live in a commercial civilization, defined by materialism, which discriminates more against the poor than against the prostitute. Women who seem particularly mean-spirited towards prostitutes are usually those who do not benefit from this materialism, and don't receive romantic attention or appreciative gifts from their husbands.

An acquaintance of mine, Ling Ling, recently migrated to Hong Kong from mainland China. She brags about her three boyfriends there who, while not married to her, still give her a sense of security. One of them is an old man with no time or energy who sees her every two weeks, while providing her with a monthly allowance of US$2,500.

Another acquaintance, Wanda, is ostensibly a ballet dancer. Despite Wanda's lack of success as a dancer, her mother is always boasting about her daughter's ability and ambition. Wanda's true ambitions seem directed elsewhere. She only picks wealthy prospects. Client A covers the cost of overseas study for both her brother and sister, B supplies her with fashionable clothes, C takes her to exclusive clubs, and D has bought her a yacht. Wanda may not be that pretty, but she seems to have the power to engender competitive jealousy. Being seen with A increases her desirability in the eyes of B, and being seen with B makes C determined to buy her a fancy car.

I have had several relationships and I still do not have a house or a car. Hearing these stories of opportunistic girls makes me think: perhaps I am wasting my natural "chicken look".

The modern world seems ready not only to tolerate prostitutes, but to return their dignity, previously denied by thousands of years of abuse. The change in attitudes interested me sufficiently to want to investigate the reality as it exists in Hong Kong, and produce a written record.

The problem became what to write, and how? There is little reference material available about Hong Kong prostitutes, even in academic libraries. In *The History of Prostitution in Hong Kong*, Ng Ho describes the Western District of Hong Kong in the 1930s and 1940s, a time considered the age of romance. The whorehouse was then the place for rich men to show off their wealth, enabling prostitutes to live in luxury way beyond the imagination of the typical housewife. These pampered celebrity whores would often dominate their male sponsors.

British journalist Kate Whitehead recently penned *After Suzie*. (*The World of Suzie Wong* was a bestselling 1950s novel about Hong Kong prostitutes. It was adapted into the movie of the same name that helped create the Suzie Wong stereotype of the Hong Kong prostitute.) The author's materials come mainly from police files, making *After Suzie* essentially a reference work that does not contain significant character depiction.

I decided the best approach was to meet a few Suzies! With this plan in mind, I mobilised my meagre resources and set off to look at the sharp end of the business.

Fred is an executive director of a large company, and he took me to Club Bboss in Tsim Sha Tsui East for a business meeting with Mr Leung, a regular visitor to expensive hostess clubs. Mr Leung is a generous man with a good sense of humour, and he is popular with the hostesses. His hero is Zhang Wuji in the famous kung fu novel *Heroes and Heroines*. He adopted the nickname Wuji because he is so fond of the clubs where he finds his 'heroines'.

One evening, at 10:30pm, Fred led me through the grandiose lobby of Bboss, along an ornate corridor and into a huge hall decorated in French baroque style. The coffee table in the centre was as big as two king-size beds and circled by huge sofas. The only other guest present was Wuji, who was accompanied by three girls in nightgowns. Fred introduced me to a middle-aged woman in a black uniform. This was mama-san Monica of Team 98. Wuji had already told her of my intentions.

Monica looked 40, clean, neatly dressed, and gracefully mannered, putting to shame the slovenly behaviour of the three smoking hostesses. Monica's husband was the manager there, and the couple would work until the last customer left. The club's male managers had different functions. They arranged the meetings between the girls and customers, helping to make customers feel more respected. After Monica's husband had welcomed Wuji into the club, and before Fred and I arrived, Wuji had opened a super-sized bottle of XO cognac, and was happy for two girls to just sit with him while he paid for their time in full. This typically profligate expenditure ensured his sky-high popularity.

Monica did not look like the classic mama-san as often depicted in popular films. As she put it, "Movies always demonise us." She told me that the movie *Stars/Moon/Sun* was about prostitutes, and that she had worked with the producer and director to make the script commercial. I remembered the film and perhaps that had contributed towards my negative impression of the mama-san. Monica said the girls nowadays were cheap, and did not even want to spend money to dress decently. Customers did not even bother to remember their names, content just to recognise them by their dress and general appearance. This increasingly impersonal attitude over her 20-year career made her feel ashamed: the girls were not as professional as before and had no interest in making any effort to attract men. They felt that simply making themselves available was sufficient.

When I asked her how much social prejudice the girls suffered, she said there was no prejudice at all; being a hostess was perfectly all right. So I rephrased the question: "How do the girls deal with prejudice and discrimination?" This was met with a burst of laughter from Wuji, who ridiculed the notion and said, "My wife used to be a hostess, so you tell me, what prejudice do I have?"

One of the girls then said, "Customers here are quite decent and nice to us."

"Your idea is old, you are thinking of 30 years ago," added Monica's husband.

I believe many customers don't despise the girls. It is a simple transaction and both parties get what they want. My interest in the question of external prejudice led me to ask, "When the girls reveal their real work to their families and friends, what happens?"

Another girl said, "We never want to talk about it, and we don't have to, so there's not much trouble."

"Everyone watches over his privacy nowadays," said Monica's husband. "People in other trades don't talk much about what they do or where they work. Plus, these girls are not chickens. Your question is for the pimps in Mong Kok [an area of cheap clubs and brothels]."

To claim the hostesses in Club Bboss are not chickens is a fine distinction. Nothing may happen on the club premises, where the girl is a hostess only. A customer may, however, buy her time and take her outside where he deals directly with her, usually for sex transactions. Even if a hostess's time is not bought in this way, she still makes the waitress income. This means she does not have to make overt advances or tolerate groping from customers. Once taken outside, if they only went for the meal and did not accept further deals, they would become known as uncooperative and the mama-san would definitely fire them. So how is it they are not chickens?

Monica answered, "I'll give you many breathtaking stories for your book, but please don't portray the hostesses as chickens." One hostess in a revealing outfit was keen to add, "Of course we are not chickens."

Monica talked me into singing. I wanted to sing a Japanese song, so she immediately called over a girl who knew Japanese. Fred said we shouldn't call over any more girls, but Monica simply looked the other way and said he was drunk.

Then another mama-san walked in with one more girl. Fred told that mama-san the three of us did not need a fourth girl, but she pretended not to hear. This annoyed Fred and he whispered in my ear, "You must sing hard, the songs here are very expensive!"

I asked Wuji why he liked to fool around in these places. He said he found nightclubs simultaneously the most relaxing and the most exciting places to ease away the tensions and suspicions between strangers. He said striking a business deal takes at most 15 minutes, but even when a deal is secured after straight business talk, one still feels a bit upset and not so sure if it was the right decision. He claimed that if the deal took place in a nightclub, things would be completely different. Firstly, he could let the hostess make the small talk, and pretty soon, everybody would be in a relaxed and romantic mood, which greatly lowered the level of anxiety and suspicion: good for a successful deal. Once trust was built, a long-term partnership could be expected.

I joked with Wuji, "Then businesswomen should go to duck [toy boy] houses." Fred cut in, "Theoretically you are correct, but this is a man's world."

Wuji told me he was a man with a tremendous need for love, and there were many lovely girls in the nightclubs, so he was always crazily in love. Gradually, the wine went to my head, and a hostess with a cigarette was singing a pop song about love and hate. The room was filled with loud music and erotic expectation. The men were feeling the girls' thighs. The singing hostess imbued the sentimental lyrics of the cheap song with surprising power, enough for the sugary tune to make me experience the intended romantic yearning. I finally understood Wuji's comments about relaxation, excitement, and crazy love. At that moment, in that company, the sensations were infectious and I felt that I too could succumb.

At 2:20 in the morning, the bill of HK$15,000 (US$2,000) arrived. I was shocked, but Wuji paid up calmly, saying it was perfectly reasonable for the wine and four girls' working time. I knew I would never again be able to afford meeting nightclub hostesses at their place of work!

I hopped into a cab alone, still missing the sexual ambience. The driver asked me: "Just knocked off? How is business going?" He took me to be a hostess. I was so embarrassed that I immediately made up a story. This made me feel guilty, because deep in my heart I was experiencing a subtle sympathy for the hostesses who claim they are not chickens.

My friend Ray is a painter. He introduced me to a great beauty from Dalian, who he had met in a nightclub. She told me she had come to Hong Kong to visit her relatives and planned to stay for half a year. Living in Tsim Sha Tsui, an area with many hostess clubs, she slept during the day and went out at night. When people made sexual jokes, she would put on the naive look of a virgin. Obviously she did not want me to find out about her business. Seeing she wanted to make friends, however, I took her out to lunch and got straight to the point. I asked whether she could recommend a hooker for my interview. Her answer was a firm "No".

After drawing a blank with Ray's lady from Dalian, I needed another plan to find a genuine chicken.

There was a news report about 'Purple Vine' – an NGO fighting for sex workers' rights, founded by a Ms Yip, a former member of a labour union.

The aim of Purple Vine was to form the first sex workers' union in Hong Kong. I decided I must meet Ms Yip. Through three introductions, I finally managed to arrange a meeting in a café. She greeted me aggressively with "What's so special about prostitutes that you want to write about them?"

While I was struggling for a quick answer, she said seriously, "If you want to write about the miserable life of the prostitute, I'd suggest you quit, all hooker literature is the same old shit."

I was excited to find she shared my opinion. Ms Yip continued in a bitter tone: "If sex workers' rights as promoted by feminists are accepted, will society one day treat sex workers just like sales assistants in department stores?"

I tried to make her feel that I was on her side. "When sex workers enjoy human rights, they won't have to go to the underworld for protection or rely on drugs as an escape. If society can accept prostitutes as a permanent phenomenon, then why not deal with it, and provide them legal protection? Governments can raise tax from their activities and they can be offered sex education, medical treatment and welfare facilities."

My answer didn't please Ms Yip. Her tone was still hard: "Nothing new in your talk. Churchgoers will attack you for violating family values."

"Prostitutes have always coexisted with the marriage system and they have never challenged family values," I replied.

Ms Yip continued, "We advocates of sex worker rights only want to stress that prostitution is just another type of work. Our opponents say prostitution is like drug trafficking, which is forbidden in a healthy society. How do you reply to that? From the feminist perspective, it's an even more complex picture. There are many schools of feminist ideology, and some say if prostitution was legalised, women would be reduced to the status of a commodity for consumption by men, and this would enhance the rule of patriarchy. How will your book deal with these charges?" I had no immediate reply.

She continued to lecture me: "A few months' research and you will only come up with a cheap shot like a new *Suzie Wong*."

I accepted this might be true and pleaded with her to introduce me to her sex worker members in order to help me understand. She would not help, telling me to look for them on the street. "They won't eat you alive. Never look down upon them."

Later, several sociologists told me that Ms Yip was trying to monopolise the media exposure of Hong Kong sex workers. Her sex workers' union had only a few members, mainly aged women, the majority of whom were humanitarian journalists. The union membership included only two or three old, retired prostitutes.

I had never expected it to be so difficult to find sex workers who would speak for themselves in Hong Kong – a place filled with chickens and ducks. I was now so fascinated by this confusion of thinking around the subject of prostitutes' rights that I became even more determined. The confusion only served to validate my initial impulse to interview, observe, think and write. It was necessary to escape from the maze of preconceptions and pundits with their eyes wide shut.

Even today, I cannot understand why I felt so strongly. I was not an academic researcher, nor did I receive any advance payment from a publisher. I was just someone whose imagination had been captured, and who could spend some time writing after work. That year, 1999, I spent all my spare time, and some personal savings, on the streets of Hong Kong interviewing nearly 50 hookers, toy boys, transsexual sex workers, mama-sans and brothel owners.

In the beginning, I was depressed by my small budget. I had no money to visit premises offering sex services, nor could I afford to interview sex workers by paying for their time.

Ironically, I would like to thank those who charged me extra for giving interviews. These sex workers, with whom I first managed to make contact, were on the shortlist of informants available to professional journalists. The journalists had bigger budgets than I did, and worked against deadlines. The sex worker interviewees had learned that the journalists, who paid well, wanted colourful stories. They elaborated and embroidered accordingly. Reading the small body of literature available, certain accounts became strangely familiar. It was a case of sex workers selling their own urban legends as another form of prostitution.

My lack of funds meant I was not a victim of these apocryphal accounts and had to devote more time to making friends with sex workers rather than treating them merely as paid interview subjects. Although it was a much slower process, I gained genuine insights into real lives. My patience rewarded me with material quite different from commercial journalism, which is often quickly written against deadlines and full of sensational accounts designed to increase newspaper circulation.

Not being a hooker myself, how can I speak authentically? In Taiwan, a postgraduate wrote her dissertation *18 Hostesses* based on her decision to become a real-life hooker for the purpose of research. That's some book to read!

Annabel Chong is perhaps the most notorious example of research taken to the extreme. Curiosity and notions of empowerment eventually led this Singaporean gender studies student to engage in an organised gang bang, during which she had sex with 251 men in ten hours.

Despite these exploits, I believe the non-hooker perspective has its own edge. Various forms of commercial sex permeate society. Hong Kong is no different and has a huge variety of sex businesses including services to suit the most freakish and outlandish of tastes. Even if I did try to prostitute myself, I would likely end up digging my own tiny, burning pit of shame. Could my potentially narrow vision provide a valuable contribution to understanding the sex industry?

The original Chinese-language version of *Whispers and Moans* was serialised in Hong Kong's *Literary Century* magazine during 2000 and 2001. It was published as a book in 2002 and both editions sold out. The Japanese version came out in 2003, with further good sales. A version in simplified Chinese characters for the mainland was blocked by the Central Bureau of Censorship in Beijing in 2003. The official reason for prohibiting its publication in mainland China was that it contained too many 'unhealthy' words (any description of sexuality is regarded as unhealthy in China). The real reason for rejection was the reform to the Marriage Law of 2002, which aimed to restore family moral values in China. Under this new law, any literature on affairs outside marriage is regarded as 'controversial' or 'spiritual pollution'. A book about sex workers stood little chance of acceptance.

On the other hand, the discussions opened in *Whispers and Moans* have been widely carried on in mainland China through a movie of the same title, directed by Herman Yau and scripted by myself. With a social realist approach, the movie dramatizes many of the true case studies in this book to portray typical characters found in the sex industry. Such a movie certainly cannot be approved by the film censors of the People's Republic, and thus cannot be distributed within China.

However, thanks to the availability of pirated DVDs and online video clips, it was not long before a heated discussion of the movie *Whispers and Moans* ensued on thousands of blogs and websites across China. Surprisingly, many of these web reviews were written by social workers, educators, public servants of family planning centres, and of course movie lovers, who shared the same sentiments and concerns about sex workers with my filmmaking colleagues. We were particularly surprised that some viewers on the mainland spent precious time translating the Cantonese dialogue of the movie into Putonghua, the national common language, and posted the translation on websites to help other mainland audiences understand the movie.

In this English-language edition of *Whispers and Moans*, I remain grateful for my original, naive impulse, without which I would never have found the determination to finish the book. I have continued to observe events and changes in the Hong Kong sex industry, and have come to see the characters in this book as more complex, and much more real.

In 2008, *Whispers and Moans Part II* was produced by the same group of filmmakers, with the subtitle *True Women For Sale*. The script of *Part II* was developed from two individual stories told in this book: Chapter 6 and Chapter 9. The second film was a huge success, not only gaining more audience support in mainland China through pirated DVDs, but also being selected as the opening movie of the 2008 Asian Film Festival, and winning Best Actress at the Golden Horse Film Festival, Asia's most important film awards ceremony.

Since then, film producers have often asked me to write a Part III screenplay, even though there are few stories in *Whispers and Moans* left to dramatize. One producer hoped to encourage me with a larger budget which would promise bigger success. But while his marketing plan was convincing, I cannot promise a Part III. I did the laborious research as a naive writer before I became an anthropologist. Now I know exactly how much additional fieldwork in the sex trade I would need to do before completing a realistic third screenplay. I just do not have the courage to do that hard work over again.

This book focuses on how Hong Kong prostitutes deal with the ruthless competition provided by mainland Chinese girls and manage to survive. Prostitutes from mainland China are increasingly encountered in cosmopolitan cities such as Tokyo, Paris, New York and London. The implications of this work are therefore not limited solely to Hong Kong society, but provide an insight into the global sex industry.

# 2

## STREET LIFE

The Catholic women's group Blue Bird was established in 1983, with the mission to love and care for prostitutes so that one day they might stand up for their own rights like any other professionals. Blue Bird social workers have found it difficult to break into the prostitutes' world. Street hookers, however, are easy targets as they are the most easily visible. This allows social workers to approach them, and sometimes, when business is slow, the girls choose to pour out their hearts to pass the time. The social workers also take the opportunity to distribute pamphlets about sexually transmitted diseases, condoms, and basic legal advice. Only after years of painstaking effort have Blue Bird's social workers gained a little trust from the prostitutes.

At first, many street hookers took Blue Bird to be a charity organisation, so they would ask for loans. When they could not get the money, they thought it was because the social workers did not believe their tales of woe, so they would elaborate their misery and say anything they could think of to get some reaction. When there was still no money forthcoming, their reaction would be: "What the fuck is your game? What are you here for?" The more polite ones would say: "We've seen more problems than you've had hot dinners, so how can you help us? You don't give us a cent, yet you say you are here to help."

A street hooker was once pursued by creditors. The creditors went to the Blue Bird office and asked staff if they would loan their client the money. If not, they said, she'd be dead, in which case she may as well throw herself out of the office window. The creditors did not realise that Blue Bird pays just two of their social workers a low salary, and the remainder are volunteers. The organisation is run by well-intentioned people who have sacrificed their pursuit of a middle-class lifestyle. Even if the creditors had tortured the impecunious prostitute right there in the office, Blue Bird simply could not produce the money.

Although Blue Bird accepted my application to be a voluntary worker, secretary-general Sister Anita required me to finish the full training course before allowing me to contact street hookers. I learned much from the training, and corrected my habit of asking people "What do you do for a living?" when meeting them for the first time.

A person's value does not lie in their profession. No one has the right to persuade prostitutes to change their job; this is discrimination. Comfortably middle-class, educated women may advocate the notion that women will not meet discrimination if they understand self-respect, and if pushed they may respond with the cold logic of "If I can do it, then you can too." This argument is valid up to a point but it overlooks women who may not have the prerequisite self-confidence.

Aids research indicates that prostitutes and their customers are well aware of the risks, so demanding that a prostitute uses condoms applies another form of discrimination. The demand clearly separates her from women with whom one might have a loving and romantic relationship. A mistress is generally kept on the basis she represents an alternative wife. If she insists on using condoms, she spoils the image of the commodity she is striving to sell.

Official anti-vice campaigns also apply pressure to avoid condom usage. If a condom is found in a woman's handbag, it will be submitted in court as evidence of prostitution. This places hookers under pressure to give up safe sex. This is also a major problem in mainland China.

Street hookers can be seen scattered along the pavements of Yau Ma Tei, Sham Shui Po, Tsuen Wan, Yuen Long and Tuen Mun like lost souls maintaining a lonely vigil. Street walking involves only three parties: the customer, the girl, and the owner of a clock room, which is rented by the hour. There is no pimp or gangster involved and so there are rarely any commission charges. Usually, the prostitute and the clock room owner have a long-term partnership, so there may be an arrangement where she has a reserved room. Before the last financial crisis, the street prostitute would offer a set course of services for HK$400-450. Since the economic recession in 1998, and severely increased competition, the set price is now down to HK$200. Although the prices are low, street hookers are free to start and finish working whenever they like and are free to choose their customers. Many high-class hookers working in clubs, who are better paid, envy this freestyle prostitution.

The two biggest obstacles for Hong Kong street hookers are the small size of Hong Kong, which means being seen by unsuspecting acquaintances is almost inevitable, effectively announcing to them "I'm a low-class hooker"; and the likelihood of being arrested and charged with 'seducing others for an indecent act'. Although the penalty is light, even a short stretch in a women's prison is hardly a sweet experience.

The typical Hong Kong streetwalker is an ageing prostitute who has been unable to quit the profession. Many have problems of drug addiction and gambling, and debts. Since the financial crisis in 1998, this community has been subject to an influx of new blood.

Many newcomers are housewives who work on the street dressed as if out shopping. Customers, however, seem able to distinguish these women from the genuine shopper.

Thai women have also become more noticeable. Normally, they only try work on the street when they can speak a little Cantonese, and in order to avoid noisy and troublesome customers they are likely to hire a pimp or a bodyguard as a partner.

Young girls have also become much more noticeable. They find nightclub prostitution too constrained by rules and dislike the rigid work schedule. Even the most popular club hostess can only strike one deal a day, while the street girls can operate with much more flexibility. Young street girls often have a cavalier attitude and ignore the unwritten turf codes. An old hooker told me that she started to panic after a long dry spell. To fight back, she gathered a group of older hookers together and demanded the young newcomers give them all the money they had made by trespassing on their turf. The youngsters did not hand over any money, but promised to stay away in future.

Another source of competition is ladyboys, or transsexuals. Transsexual friends have told me that "90% of ladyboys are prostitutes." Ladyboys like to show off their female personas. Their particular appetite for street work provides constant reinforcement of their attractiveness to men. Very few ladyboys have undergone gender reassignment surgery, but most have had surgery to reduce the prominence of their Adam's apples.

Girls with various levels of learning disability are also working on the streets. They attract sufficient customers to keep working because, anecdotally, they do whatever they are asked.

The major source of competition is women from mainland China. They have flourished on Hong Kong streets, providing a cut-price paradise for customers and creating a nightmare for local hookers.

Hong Kong locals call them northern girls. They have a reputation for being tough and able to look after themselves without needing help from anyone else. Despite this, their weakness is their entry visa, which lasts for three months if they are visiting, but only one month if they work. Some northern girls have visited Hong Kong so often that alert immigration officers give visas for one week only. The shorter the visa, the harder the girls must work. Highly priced northern girls usually take temporary work in top-class nightclubs and karaoke lounges, saving their spare time for streetwalking or working the hotel lobbies in the east section of Tsim Sha Tsui.

Northern girls play an important role in Hong Kong's sex industry. Blue Bird, Purple Vine and other NGOs providing social welfare are aware of them but find it virtually impossible to make contact. The suspicious girls take the social workers to be police officers, and run for cover the moment they are approached by a smiling woman.

Newly migrated Miss Hu was from Hubei province and was often seen in shorts and a T-shirt. She carved out a street corner in Yau Ma Tei as her territory. Miss Hu was pleasingly full-figured with clear, fair skin, which is highly prized. She liked to give me her family gossip. Lately, it seemed, her daughter thought there was a ghost in their house, so she would burn paper money every day for good luck. Most recently, her daughter had asked: "What if my arm was broken? What if I went blind?" Miss Hu was concerned that her daughter had a mental illness, but the child psychiatrist said she was fine.

I said, "Maybe your daughter wants your attention." Miss Hu snapped a response: "I've got to hang around here for a whole day to make just a few deals. How can I have time for her bullshit?" I asked how long she had been standing out there. She said there had been no work for a long time. I said, "If you've got no business anyway, why not go home and see your daughter?" Again, her temper showed: "Business is suffering; how can I be in the right mood for baby-sitting?" She continued: "I'm getting old. I've only got a few years left, I've got to make good use of them."

Quite unexpectedly, my Blue Bird colleague and I ran into a 20-year-old street hooker who told us her name was Ah Mei. Despite the cold weather, she would always wait on the dark street corner in a brief miniskirt. Each time we met, she would greet us first: "I heard you've come to help us, can you find me a job? I used to work in a bakery."

I would eventually arrange an interview for her, but customers asking her prices would always be interrupting our conversations. For a decent looking customer, her price was HK$300; if the customer looked rough or too old, she'd charge HK$350. It was a good deal and customers would rarely bargain with her. Dangling a key from her hand, Ah Mei would lead the customer to a clock room in a nearby building. Within 15 minutes, the customer would come down, followed by Ah Mei brushing her hair. Ah Mei had many regular patrons who complained about her changing locations and irregular hours, which made it hard to find her. They tried asking for her mobile number, but Ah Mei always claimed her mobile could only make outgoing calls.

When I met her again, I told her that a certain bakery was recruiting, but I could not reach her because I didn't have her mobile number. When I asked for it, she used the same excuse, that she could only make outgoing calls. Then, a customer came by. After business was done, she came down to see me still waiting. As if we had not spoken previously, she started: "I used to sell bread, can you get me a job in a bakery?"

A street hooker from northeast China dropped her defences and chatted with me. She said she made frequent visits to Hong Kong, usually for durations of seven days. She had friends running clock hotels in Hong Kong, so she didn't need to pay house rent, and would spend the night with customers. Working in Hong Kong gave her better prices and the police treatment was less harsh than on the mainland. If she was caught, the worst thing that could happen was being repatriated. In addition, Hong Kong police would never confiscate her prostitution earnings.

Ah Kwan looked to be only in her 30s, and she would talk endlessly about her boyfriend. It was one story after another, all about her crazy love for this remarkable boyfriend who took wonderful care of her. Then she would emphasise that for such a lovely man, she would do anything. Her income, unfortunately, had to support the drug habits of two addicts, which is nothing unusual and is a stereotype among street hookers. Her story is memorable because the boyfriend with whom she was so besotted was 70 years old.

Gaining age and weight, Ah Fung would sit alone by the roadside with a large bag of bubble wrap. She would absent-mindedly pop the bubbles to pass the time. When she met us, she would give us some of the bubble wrap so we could all pop the bubbles together. Only when the bubbles were exhausted would she talk to us. Ah Fung hated young customers the most because they didn't like using condoms. Her favourites were older men who were less likely to argue with her.

Once, the famous Hong Kong movie director Ann Hui and I went to a well-known hooker street in Sham Shui Po to collect ladyboy material. Ah Fung was excited when she recognised Ann: "I have many excellent stories. I'll tell you all. It's for free. Just leave me your number."

I have no appetite for self-promoted stories, but Ann didn't mind leaving Ah Fung her number. Two weeks later, she spared an afternoon to have tea with Ah Fung to ask about the relationship between street hookers and ladyboys, but Ah Fung started with a few dirty jokes, which Ann found hilarious. Ah Fung had great fun telling jokes and Ann had an afternoon of belly laughs. Ah Fung didn't charge Ann for the jokes, she only hoped that they would play a role in her movies.

At Lung Wah Theatre in Tsuen Wan, we ran into a middle-aged new migrant, who immediately took us to be government agents of some description. She screamed at us that the police had already arrested her six times that month. "There's no place to hook any more. Sham Shui Po, Yau Ma Tei and Mongkok are bursting with girls, and so I had to come to Tsuen Wan to try my luck. Just this month, I spent HK$100,000 on a lawsuit."

It was a chilling figure. How many customers did she have to receive to cover such legal fees? Later, my volunteer colleagues told me she was well off, having already finished paying the mortgage instalments for several houses.

Ah Ching was a skeletal figure with grey, sepulchral features. She walked with an uncanny gliding motion, like an apparition floating on water. She said that night-shift taxi drivers often took her to be a ghost; apparently, they would pull over in front of her and then flee after taking a closer look. Whenever she met us, she would narrow her eyes into a sad look and complain about her boyfriend's mischief. She was extremely generous in giving her love and began prostitution to pay back her first boyfriend's debt. She started taking drugs to win her second boyfriend's favour, and spent half a year in jail for taking the blame for charges against her third boyfriend of harbouring drugs. Most recently, she was going to jail again for her fourth boyfriend, but he was leaving her again. She begged him on bended knees to stay, and even offered him money, but nothing could move him.

Ah Sau had mild cerebral palsy, but was not sufficiently disabled to live in the health centre, to which her family would take her every day. With time, this became a troublesome chore for the family. Ah Sau's best friend was a street hooker called Ah Siu. Whenever I met Ah Sau in Sham Shui Po, I would see Ah Siu too.

Ah Sau told me that Ah Siu was very nice to her, buying her cigarettes every day. She liked smoking. Ah Siu would dress her up, help watch over her money, and even pass her own customers to Ah Sau. I was tempted to ask Ah Sau if she thought she was being swindled out of her earnings. I later heard that somebody else had asked the same question, resulting in Ah Sau receiving a good scolding from Ah Siu, who felt misunderstood. Ah Sau didn't feel sorry at all and was not in the least worried about being exploited. Ah Siu said if she did not help Ah Sau collect the money, would customers be honest enough to pay a disabled girl? Furthermore, if she did take any of Ah Sau's money it was not for nothing. After all, she reasoned, she was looking after Ah Sau's daily life, and even had to feed her and wipe her after using the toilet.

Ah Chai was an old hooker with a rough appearance and a vacant expression, living on a monthly HK$1,000 of government aid, which only paid for a couple of fixes of heroin. She had a tense relationship with her family, and as she could not afford anywhere of her own, she had to live in a shelter for the homeless. When she had no business, she would go without food. When it was cold, she worried about having nothing warm to wear and would curse the ill-fitting clothes distributed by the Salvation Army as being useless.

Whenever she met us, she would whisper: "Could you buy me lunch?" Sometimes she asked me: "When are you coming to interview me? I won't charge you much. I'll tell you anything. Anything you want to hear." I bought her lunch, and through a mouthful of food, she began her version of the two major problems facing local street hookers.

Many women fall into the downcast life of a street hooker because of a drug problem. Ah Chai had been to over a dozen drug rehabilitation centres all over Hong Kong, and she could remember which ones preached Jesus, which ones talked about Buddha, and which ones had good-tempered social workers. Each time she voluntarily agreed to stay in a centre she found the withdrawal process tough, yet each time she left she would be straight back on the street, back to prostitution and drugs. Social workers at the drug rehabilitation centres told me that their success rate among Hong Kong women was almost zero, but there are abundant examples of male junkies cleaning up and never looking back. Our male-dominated culture views men determined to give up drugs for self-salvation as heroes. For a female addict, the initial fall is perceived to be from a greater height and she finds it much harder to rebuild her life. Evidence suggests that even after a successful rehabilitation, a prostitute may only find full acceptance among her lifelong female junkie friends. The second time around, if sent to prison for drug taking or prostitution, her forehead will be forever marked with the words 'junkie, hooker, and prisoner'.

The second major problem is the arrival of northern girls. Visiting mainland hookers have devastated the local sex market. Facing the young, pretty, inexpensive northern girls, who are willing to accept any sex variation, the local girls, especially street hookers, are filled with rage and frustration. Ah Chai said: "Recently, I've been waiting around on the street for nothing. It can't be helped. Since the northern girls marched in, we all have to starve."

It was an early autumn evening and we were chatting with girls on the street in Sham Shui Po. The young girls teased us: "Any gifts for us?" We were delivering only condoms when a dozen police officers surrounded us, yelling: "ID check! ID check!" I was taken aside and questioned alone by a plain-clothes policeman: "Don't lie to me, how long have you been standing here?"

I said, being honest, "A couple of minutes."

"Don't try and fool me! Where did you stand before?" "Before? I have stood in many places." I suddenly realised that he had mistaken me for a hooker. I was about to explain when he adopted a sharper tone: "I'll ask you one more time, which street do you normally stand on?"

I was now feeling anxious and disorientated. "Which street? How can I remember? There are so many streets in Hong Kong. I have stood on all of them." He was infuriated: "I warn you, stop playing games! Where are you from? Who are you working with? Who is your boss?"

I could take this interrogation no more and wanted to call my colleagues so they could explain, but the officer stopped me: "You are under separate questioning; you can't call anybody!" The situation overwhelmed me and I was barely coherent.

When the police found out we were not hookers, they immediately turned on the charm and apologised profusely. We were all women, but with different labels. We were no longer 'street hookers' but 'good women'. Different labels received completely different treatment from the police. An accidental misunderstanding had scared me senseless – it was extremely hard for me to imagine how street hookers dealt with this type of interrogation on a daily basis.

# 3

## A WOMAN OF HER OWN MAKING

We are all labelled 'male' or 'female' as soon as we enter the world. Everyone, family and outsiders alike, then expects us to live according to these labels as both children and adults. As a result, many transsexuals grow up confused and isolated, deeply ashamed of who and what they are. They may try to hide their feelings, hoping they will go away, living unfulfilled lives of great unhappiness. Transsexuals are often rejected by family and friends. They may face prejudice and discrimination, particularly in employment, where they find it hard to get a job or achieve promotion. In Hong Kong, they cannot currently change their legal status. For many, even those whose partners accept them for who they are, marriage is impossible. Living socially isolated lives, they often feel depressed, helpless, and suicidal. Compared with other Asian countries, Hong Kong can be a particularly tough place for transsexuals, and this aggravates the tendency towards suicide.

Joey has a delicate face with beautiful hair tumbling onto her shoulders. Despite being a little overdone, immaculate make-up gives her a radiant appearance. She has looks that could melt your soul. Perfectly manicured hands with elegant fingernails rest on her lap and draw attention to her brief skirt and long, silken thighs. The collar of her black velvet top opens wide to reveal a deep cleavage between firm, snow-white breasts. Stunning enough, but at six feet tall the effect is utterly devastating.

Joey stands out among the street hookers at Sham Shui Po. Even her broad torso and toned arms do not detract from her feminine charm. One cannot help but gaze upon this Amazon whose beauty is truly hypnotic.

The first time I saw her, I could not resist the desire to talk to her. As I approached, I was taken aside and asked to produce my ID card by a police officer who obviously mistook my intentions. I was interrogated like a suspect while other policemen yelled at other hookers to move on. Despite the police presence, no one disturbed Joey; she calmly glanced around, rose slowly from her seat and then gently strutted away. Her breathtaking beauty cut a swathe through bystanders, distracting everybody. Even the policemen paused for a moment to steal a glance before resuming their duties.

At Yau Ma Tei I met Sally. She was holding a soft drink, wearing cheap clothes and faux jewellery. She swayed her hips, stuck out her fake breasts and played the coquette. She shot smiles at anybody and everybody, and pranced along the filthy street as if it was her stage.

Although her face had coarse features, and the Adam's apple was obvious, her self-indulgence was still quite touching. Each time I met her, she would flip her dainty fingers and greet me warmly with a "Hi", then walk on with her flirty catwalk stroll. She always seemed to be in a rush and I never managed to chat with her, except overhearing her say to another transsexual: "Men are so dumb. Why pay me all that money just for a quick hand job. I could understand if they wanted something more interesting or if I was helping them jerk off a whole gang of studs. Then they might get value!"

Yau Ma Tei had several other transsexual hookers following the same slightly too feminine dress code. Instead of waiting quietly on the street like other hookers, their technique was to promote themselves aggressively: "Like to know me, sir? You'll never forget me." One day, a street hooker in Tsuen Wan told me: "We used to have a truce with the ladyboys, each guarding our own turf, but now they snatch any business they can. They don't even tell their customers they've got no pussy. They deserve a good beating."

In the heterosexual world, the sexes are polarised: men are men and women are women. Those with obscure gender features survive in their own tiny space. Friends of a girl from a liberal Singaporean family supported the girl's sister through reassignment surgery to solve her gender identity crisis. However, the whole family found itself suffering a gender identity crisis. The family struggled hard to erase memories of the erstwhile sister in order to adapt to the new brother.

A friend at Hong Kong University who has studied transsexual issues said: "Transsexuals are accepted in Southeast Asia, but in Hong Kong they are literally called 'ladyboy monsters', and most Hong Kong transsexuals are suicidal." In 2004, the media reported that four transsexuals had committed suicide in Hong Kong. The headlines exploited the deaths and used words like 'perversion' and 'sickness' to sell more copies.

Fanny signed a contract to work for a nightclub as a madam, but she didn't have enough hostesses and began to think of recruiting some of the younger street hookers working in Sham Shui Po. One night, she asked me to go to Sham Shui Po with her to find some girls. While strolling around, she noticed the beautiful Joey. She approached Joey and peppered her with questions like: How much do you make each day? Do you want to work in a nightclub? Have you ever fancied girls? Have you had surgery? Are you taking hormone injections? Giving nothing away, the streetwise Joey managed to avoid giving direct answers, leaving us none the wiser.

During that recruiting trip, Fanny tried hard but found no likely girls. She could not stop thinking of Joey. Her own experiences as a prostitute told her that Joey must have suffered unthinkable misery, so she forgave her the vague responses to her questions. The next day, she treated Joey to drinks and assured her: "I understand your misgivings about working in a nightclub, with the risk of being humiliated by the hostesses and bullied by the customers. Please accept this treat in a spirit of goodwill."

A traffic jam made me ten minutes late for my appointment with Joey that had been arranged by Fanny, who had called me very early in the morning to urge me: "Don't arrive early and don't be late. Bring some small gifts. You must pay an interview fee. Don't ask embarrassing questions, they are very sensitive." With her exhortations in mind, I rushed to the meeting with a heavy heart.

As if waiting for a customer, Joey was sitting in the lobby of a large building, staring into the middle distance with a vacant expression. She casually waited for me to finish my apology for being late, then stood up and led me into a nearby café.

Joey was born in Shanghai in 1970. As a child at elementary school, she liked colourful clothes, playing with dolls, looking in the mirror, and using red paper cut-outs as lipstick. When she was ten years old, one boy in her class was especially tender to her and she ached to spend every minute with him. Two years later, her family migrated to Hong Kong. Being tall for her age at middle school, she was more comfortable hanging out with older pupils, smoking, drinking, dancing and taking ecstasy. Her parents were always fighting and their marriage ended in divorce, after which they had no time or energy to care for Joey's physical and mental wellbeing.

Perhaps in an attempt to draw attention not provided by her parents, Joey liked to dress up very girlishly to attract people's looks on the street. The attention thrilled her but the cost of clothes to maintain her new persona was high. At 14, men in discos would try to pick her up, and she soon realised that her body could be a source of income if she was willing to submit to anal sex. Each time she sold herself, she enjoyed unspeakable satisfaction. She didn't think of herself as homosexual as she neither liked penetration nor felt excitement at the sight of a penis.

The excitement for her came from the pickup, as it affirmed her charm and attractiveness. A heterosexual customer proved she was equal to a real woman in terms of glamour and female beauty. She liked to serve customers and maintained a professional approach. Although she never liked anal sex, she would nonetheless acquiesce and guarantee satisfaction.

Having a penis is associated with fear of penetration, which symbolises being conquered, dominated, and even ravished. This is symptomatic of male territorial behaviour, which encourages defence against any other male that threatens an invasion of territory, personal space or body. Joey accepted her male genitals and retained an element of maleness in that when dressed as a man, she would not let even the finest men enjoy her anally, as she considered it a humiliation. Even when in women's clothes, although professionally available, she still would not let a coarse or crude male customer violate her just for a wad of cash.

Surrounded by friends who liked to socialise with her, Joey always needed cash. She learned not to let customers pick her, but to aggressively provoke, attract and control the customers she accepted. In a sex deal, she would choose an appropriate sexual activity depending on whether she was dressed as a man or a woman. She took care to maintain her notions of male dignity while acknowledging her feminine qualities. As a man, Joey was a dignified gigolo who offered only blowjobs, giving the customer the experience of alternating mouthfuls of ice, hot tea and soda water. Anal sex was definitely not on offer from Joey's male incarnation.

After leaving school, Joey had an active social life, with easily made money easily spent. She gathered around her a bunch of liberal friends who did not care if she was male or female, or if she was physically different; they just wanted fun, and everybody wanted ecstasy. Joey used ecstasy for two years, and during this period still did not know if she was gay or a woman in a man's body. Along the way, in addition to learning how to dress well and tastefully, she discovered her singing talent. In a bar band in Wan Chai, Joey rose from a chorus singer to the lead vocals, singing melancholy songs in glamorous dresses. She played the role of classic torch singer to perfection.

During puberty, Joey experienced a nocturnal emission. She was not fond of masturbation. Her penis grew extremely slowly, completely out of proportion to her large body size, and she had plump, rounded buttocks and smooth skin. Before falling asleep, she would fantasise about kissing a handsome boy as a girl. During her teenage years, before Hello Kitty, she would delight in finding pink, dainty, girlish toys.

A clinical diagnosis labelled her as having 'anaemic transsexualism'. This unhelpful term is now replaced by the general description of gender dysphoria, or gender identity disorder, which is applied to conditions where an individual feels they do not match the gender of their physical body. The description 'transgendered' also applies. The individual may display a wide range of behaviours. Transsexualism is associated with a persistent desire to change the body to match the mind, and may be resolved by counselling or therapy to assist in dealing with feelings of confusion and discomfort. Many transsexuals feel the only solution is gender reassignment surgery.

In a traditional society where men are men and women are women, gender confusion can cause revulsion in particularly conservative individuals. People supposing themselves to be normal may grimace, and comment to others: "Is it a man or a woman?" After a cursory appraisal they would answer their own question: a ladyboy! This term transcends the gender boundaries, indicating neither a man nor a woman, but an uncomfortable union of both; something 'other' that confounds the normal human tendency to analyse new information by forcing it into existing pigeonholes.

Like any teenager, Joey was eager to seek group identity by finding a way to fit in. However, her gender dysphoria sapped her vigour. Every day, Joey would ponder the same question: to be a boy or a girl? If she dressed as a man, the decision would go against her will and she would suffer self-disgust; if she dressed as a woman, it would contradict her physiology and Joey would despise herself equally. Ultimately, Joey would be neither a man nor a woman. She was in an impossible position. She could not even figure out the most basic of situations: How to enter a public restroom? How to date? How to choose a profession? How to tick the gender box on the immigration form? How to live the rest of her life?

Even if the gender issue were completely ignored by the world at large, those who have gender dysphoria would still tend towards feelings of guilt, self-loathing, self-blame and self-punishment. Serious depression may develop, eventually leading to suicide. Joey did not know that the medical world understood her suicidal feelings. Her way out was to take ecstasy. When the high wore off, she would remember her family and how her parents felt sorry for her. Her sense of guilt would return, only to be expunged by another hit of ecstasy.

One day, Tsoi told Joey: "You are the one woman for me. You are the love of my life!" Earnest passion burned in his eyes and vaporised the last drop of male hormone in Joey's body. This was her big day. She fell in love and accepted the lady in her ladyboy identity. Joey's remarried mother said: "Whether you are a son or a daughter, or neither, you are still my baby."

Joey threw away her padded bras and began to take female hormone injections. Her breasts and hips gradually swelled and the tiresome penis shrank away. She finally began to be proud of her female identity.

Tsoi dumped his pretty girlfriend, a gentle beauty who was living with him, in order to be with Joey. In return, Joey drew out all her savings from selling sexual favours in order to cover Tsoi's gambling debts. At first, they were inseparable. Then, Tsoi took her to a gambling house where he became involved in a prolonged session that lasted several days and nights. Before Joey could enjoy the taste of a man's real love, Tsoi had to run away from loan sharks. She cashed in all her valuables, but Tsoi said it was not enough. Joey was worried that he would borrow money from his ex-girlfriend, and she would never let him lose face like that. He was her lover, and paying back his debt was her duty alone; no business of the ex-girlfriend.

Joey went to her stepfather's house, gathered up all her mother's cash and jewellery into a cotton bag and handed them over to Tsoi, who disappeared the next day. After three days of searching for him, Joey learned that Tsoi and his ex-girlfriend had gone to Japan for a holiday.

The confidence that had taken so long to develop was crushed in an instant. Heartbroken, she tried to end her life by slashing her wrists, but the blade was too blunt to do real harm. She waited to bleed to death, so she thought, but it took so long that she became bored and her mind began to wander. She felt that being halfway through suicide, there was nothing more to fear, so why not go the whole hog and live fully as a woman? The suicide attempt stemmed from feeling insufficiently feminine, and after all, Joey did want to be a woman. While waiting to die, she admired her striking eyes in a mirror, and the more she looked at them, the more she loved them. How could she die with such beautiful eyes?

Having survived the suicide attempt, Joey continued to practise using her eyes. With a mirror, she was able to observe her 'come hither' expression from various angles. Eventually, she developed an engaging, tender, flirtatious look she considered more seductive than that of any woman. Joey continued to sing in the bar, and sell herself to customers who were interested. Having chosen to live, she determined to live like a woman. She began to save for gender reassignment surgery but decided not to follow the other ladyboys who flocked to Thailand for the treatment. She heard that the quality of Thai surgeons was questionable and that many artificial vaginas continued to grow hair internally after the operation. Joey was going to America, and no matter how much it cost, she was going to a have a vagina capable of secretion and orgasm. She was born without an Adam's apple. In addition, her delicate, smooth skin saved her the expensive process of electrolysis, a must for many others.

Transsexual beauty Fei Cheong became a posthumous celebrity after she committed suicide. Her boyfriend also had the family name of Tsoi. When he was involved with Fei Cheong he came to hear Joey singing on two consecutive weeks.

One day, this older Tsoi told Joey: "I can't go to sleep without thinking of your soul-seizing eyes." He then whispered into her ear: "Fei Cheong has a dry hole, and it smells nothing like a woman." Hearing this, the narcissistic Joey was flattered. She opened up her heart and gave it to old Tsoi who, just like her earlier boyfriend, tricked her out of all her money, then vanished. Being dumped a second time, Joey was devastated and wanted to die. She decided that if she was going to die anyway, it didn't make much difference if it was tomorrow or next week. Waiting for death was tolerable. Eventually, the waiting saved her.

When Joey's mother and stepfather went to live in South Africa, she accompanied them, with a broken heart. In an English school in Johannesburg, she met Zhong from Guangzhou. He was a practical southerner who was working hard to save enough to buy a house and marry his fiancé from Guangzhou, who was family-minded. He had been there a few months and knew the ropes: where to buy cheap beer, which restaurants served greasy pork, which slot machines were more likely to pay out, and which public phone booth worked for free.

These two quite different characters, with very little in common, were driven together by their shared boredom and immigrant status. Zhong wanted to save on his house rent and Joey wanted to make friends and form a peer group, so they moved into one apartment. Zhong was a quick hand at housework, and was able to cook three good meals a day and be conscientious about each dish. Enjoying the good food, and the absence of chores, Joey became lazy. The house-proud Zhong had even taken over doing her laundry, including underwear, without saying a word.

One night, pretending to be drunk in order to gather nerve, he grabbed Joey's big body as if it was that of his dainty fiancé, and with all his energy revelled in penetrating his friend. The next day, having experienced sex more intensely than ever before, Zhong tucked his fiancé's picture into his suitcase and put Joey's picture up in its place. He then went to a furniture store to buy a king-size bed.

Because of the previous two heartbreaks, Joey was understandably wary of Zhong's love. She was restless, and would aimlessly wait around, dressed to kill, looking seductive and available. Zhong gave whatever he could from his income to help pay the balance for her sex-change operation. Joey, however, took the money for gambling, and when it was spent, she borrowed more. She paid back the small sums by turning tricks, leaving Zhong to settle the larger debts.

With no money at hand, Zhong coaxed his fiancé into selling their business in Guangzhou and made Joey swear to quit gambling, but as soon as the money arrived, Joey went gambling again. After his fiancé had sold off the fourth hairdressing salon, Zhong gave Joey a stern warning: "This is the last time I clear your debts. If you keep on gambling, you move out." Joey was distraught and knew this was her last chance. In tears she vowed that she'd not only stop gambling, but also stop carrying money to avoid the temptation, and that she'd work hard, save hard, and pay him back.

A gambler should never be trusted. Zhong drew cash from the bank to buy a second-hand car. His boss suddenly called him into the office, so he dropped the money at home and left. When he came back in the late evening, Joey was not there. Fearing the worst, he went to the casino. As he expected, he saw that familiar face, as impassive and alluring as ever. Just then, the ball began to roll in the roulette wheel, and the punters held their breath. The ball settled and the croupier raked in the chips.

Joey clutched at the air, her eyes nervously glancing from side to side. Frantically, she fumbled through all her pockets until she found a single chip, and tossed it onto the roulette table. Her face was now like that of a wild beast, grimacing as she waited for the kill. With this change of expression, Zhong could see no trace of her beauty, self-confidence, or dignified resolve in facing her gender confusion. Zhong was sickened and angrily said, "Come home with me right now."

Joey stared at him, puzzled, pale, and defeated like a beaten dog. She seemed to come back to her senses as she won her bet, and said: "One more round and I'll go." She quickly put down a few chips and won again, so she put down more for yet another bet. Zhong was at the limit of his endurance, and gave her a shove to urge her to go home. Joey glared at him; the defeated look had now turned into one of triumphant fury. "Fuck off! I'm winning. What are you yelling at? You want to scare my luck away?" Zhong went home alone, threw her belongings onto the street, and changed the locks.

Weighed down with a suitcase and infinite regret, Joey returned to her parents. She realised that Zhong was a real man and nothing like her previous boyfriends. She understood that even a ladyboy could find a good man. Joey repeated Zhong's name to herself over and over. She was desperate to see Zhong; she would never find a man like him ever again; she couldn't lose him. Zhong would not answer her phone calls. It was a cold rainy night, and there was a power blackout, so it was pitch dark. Her stepfather's car had broken down on his way home.

Her mother tried to stop her: "There's a blackout, there are no street lights, it's too dark!" Joey did not care; she had to see Zhong that night. Her mother gripped her: "It's an hour's walk, what happens if you run into a wild beast? There may be black guys who hate Chinese." Joey ran into the night as her mother called out: "Wait till daybreak. It's too dangerous."

Joey walked in the rain along muddy paths for two hours and arrived at Zhong's home dirty and bedraggled. Kneeling down in front of him crying, she blamed herself harshly and repeatedly, but Zhong was indifferent. Pointing to his fiancé's picture by his bedside, he said: "Too late! I've already called her to come over."

Her previous boyfriends had deceived her for money, and their behaviour could be written off as consistent with that of common cheats. This loss was more painful. It hurt her dignity, and the pain produced feelings of hatred that would otherwise have driven her on, but losing Zhong was like losing her heart and soul.

Her four years in South Africa had passed in the blink of an eye. Joey had grown comfortable with her ladyboy identity. If she wanted to be a man, Joey would dress in fashionable, casual men's clothes and visit the mens' room without hesitation. If she felt the impulse to be a woman, she'd take injections of female hormones to fill out her breasts, but she dared not go to the ladies' room for fear of trouble. Ironically, her three failed romances proved to her that she could be a woman, and gave her heart to look forward to the future. Joey decided not to stay in South Africa, which would mean dealing with issues of nationality, race and gender. She returned to Hong Kong to live in a familiar cultural environment.

Transsexuals constantly want to verify their female identity, and being a prostitute reinforces confidence in their desirability. Street hookers can strike more sex deals than hostesses in clubs, which is why, whether pretty or ugly, ladyboys always choose to be street hookers. On the street they can attract curious looks, bait whoever takes their fancy, and serve whichever customers they choose. This avoids bars and dance halls where they have less control and might have to wait on 'freaks'. It is a matter of particular pride to pick up straight customers.

On her return to Hong Kong, Joey rented an apartment in a pre-war *tong lau* building in Sham Shui Po to serve as both accommodation and a place to take customers. Apart from sleeping, she spent most of her time waiting at the street entrance to her apartment. Joey was popular, and tried not to upset her neighbours. She never lied to customers and would always strike a sex deal after telling them she had not yet had surgery. All her customers were typical men out cruising for sex, but the other street hookers did not see her as a rival. They liked her and treated her as a sister.

The local streets were filled with shabby houses, signboards, shops and food stands. It was a place for business of all kinds. Men choosing to visit the area had a personal agenda. Whenever a social worker or a charity distributed condoms in the neighbourhood, Joey would get one.

In all weather, through cool damp winters and hot steamy summers, Joey waited on the street for customers. She became a celebrity hooker in Sham Shui Po. During good times, she might receive over a dozen customers a day, at other times, perhaps only two. For each 20-minute service, she charged HK$300, which produced a reasonable income. This money was supplemented by the generous sums paid by the many reporters who came to interview her and gather material on her lifestyle.

Waiting on the street was a drag, and she broke the monotony by gambling. There were those who did not appreciate her presence. Some old men who disapproved would shoot stones at her face with catapults. These surprise attacks hospitalised her, which reduced her income. She never seemed to earn quite enough. Luckily, she had patrons from all over Hong Kong Island, Kowloon, Lantau Island and the New Territories. Some customers would come to her directly after returning from overseas, before even taking their luggage home. What made Joey most proud was that most of her customers were not freaks, but normally straight men; even gigolos, who specialised in serving female customers, would come to see her.

Keong often came to Sham Shui Po for prostitutes, and Joey aroused his curiosity. After Joey's service, Keong stopped seeing other hookers, and came to see her more frequently. Slowly, he became Joey's boyfriend, inviting her to dinner almost every day. When she was with a customer, he would wait outside, and when the customer had gone, he would buy her chicken soup.

Keong's wife became suspicious of her husband's behaviour and so she followed him to Joey's room at Sham Shui Po. She broke in and found a shocking scene. She screamed at Joey: "You fucking freak! Damn fucking freak!" Infuriated, Keong grabbed his wife by her clothes and yelled at her: "Since you followed me here, there's no need to hide any more. I want a divorce!" His stunned wife fell into a deep panic.

If it had been a female, even a worn-out, cheap hooker, she might have been able to understand, but losing her husband to a ladyboy was a gross insult. How could she call herself a woman? Joey said to Keong's wife: "I'm only doing business, and I don't want to break up your family. I have talked to Keong and urged him to think of his family responsibilities. I promise I won't maintain any special relationship with him." Hearing Joey's sincere tone, and knowing that her husband had used prostitutes for years, she relaxed slightly. She just wanted to know where she had gone wrong. Why did men have to go to prostitutes instead of taking care of their families?

Joey gave it some serious thought and said: "I sympathise with you. Men suck! Just for the sake of squirting more sperm, they will come and spend money in Sham Shui Po."

Joey was now 30 years old and had learned the lessons of her lifestyle. Reflecting on the past, her crazy romances no longer bothered her. Although she was weary of love, she still missed its bittersweet feelings and emotions. They reassured Joey of her female persona. A man's love may be shallow but its attentions comforted her, giving her the courage to be honest about her gender feelings. She believed that if she had continued living in confusion about her gender, she might still be relying on the white powder to get by, wasting her life. Alternatively, she might have married as a man and raised children, but this would have contradicted her gender feelings, and would have meant living an undercover life.

"I must have a juicy pussy," Joey confided in me. She meant one capable of secretion. Her wish was unrealistic. Because of the lack of natural secretions, a surgically created vagina requires regular artificial lubrication and douching to avoid infection and lesions.

Joey had never had an orgasm as a man; when aroused, her penis only ever became semi-tumescent. She longed to experience a female orgasm once she had undergone the operation. She had total faith that surgery would solve all her problems.

I warned Joey: "There might still be problems. Didn't Fei Cheong jump off a building after her operation?" Joey retorted: "There are more ladyboys who don't jump off buildings."

Transsexuals lust for a stable emotional life, but the assumed gender is not acknowledged by the law, so the security of marriage is not possible. Joey lit a cigarette and inhaled deeply. "All my customers have wives and kids. I've seen enough. So why would I want to get married? Legitimate marriage has no interest for me."

"So what's next for you, after becoming a woman?" I enquired. Joey replied, "Becoming a complete woman will make me whole. Then, I could do anything: I could be a model, or a singer, or keep whoring on the street." Her eyes were filled with confidence, making me feel happy for her.

For the sake of the interview, I had to ask a very difficult question. "To maintain a female physique, biological functions are compromised by constant hormone injections and medication, leading to severe damage to both your physical and mental integrity. How do you feel about that?"

"Correct, ladyboys don't live very long," Joey replied. "But what is a person if she can't be herself? I want to do what I'm able to do, and what pleases me. I am a woman!"

That was in 1999. Joey had still not had the surgery when I met her again three years later. Bad luck had prevented her from saving any money. She had suffered two more disastrous relationships, been jailed three times for harbouring drugs, and been beaten up so badly by customers that she twice had to be hospitalised. When I met her, she was crazily in love yet again, telling me she was the happiest woman in the world. Her boyfriend called her every two minutes and our conversation was ruined. Saying goodbye, she told me: "This is the last man in my life. I'll treasure him. I've really got to go."

When I met her again in 2003, she still had no money for the operation. She said the "last man" had tortured her like hell. She had finally decided that men were unreliable and so she was going to dedicate all her energy to her career. She seemed confident. She became the madam of a small nightclub in Mong Kok, winning favour with her boss and the hostesses. But after just two weeks, she suffered more bad luck. I had made a date with her in order to bring a Danish television crew to film at her nightclub. On my way there, while approaching Mong Kok, Joey called: "The boss has just fired me, saying business is bad because of SARS."

In 2004, Joey looked for me several times, saying she needed cash and was willing to reveal the secret details of her jail experiences. I recommended her to Hong Kong University scholars specialising in transsexuals. She not only failed to show up, but also switched off her phone. Two months later, she called to explain why: she had given all her money to her boyfriend, and even transferred the remaining balance on her phone card to him, so she didn't have the taxi fare for the appointment. She pleaded with us for another opportunity, which was given to her, and she stood us up again because her face was swollen from a beating by her boyfriend.

For the next few days, she called me non-stop, saying she didn't want to live any more. "Tell your transsexual study friends why Hong Kong ladyboys like to commit suicide. Because men know we crave love, they use this weakness to squeeze the last drop of blood out of us."

In one month alone in 2004, two transsexual suicides in Hong Kong were reported in the media. It is likely that more suicides are quietly taking place, without publicity; the truth about their lives concealed by families wishing to save face.

# 4

## THE LAW, GANGSTERS, AND VOLUNTEERS

The international community normally adopts one of the following three approaches to control prostitution.

First: a total ban. Like any traditional method of social control, this aims to eliminate prostitution. China used to impose a complete ban on prostitution, but even the powerful central government could not enforce the ban. Nor could it reduce the number of prostitutes. In addition, the official anti-vice campaign caused many social problems.

In the 1990s, if a suspect was found carrying a condom, the public security bureau would judge that she was a prostitute. This effectively forced sex workers into unprotected sex, with the associated health risks. Besides punishing prostitutes, the police also targeted customers. As recently as ten years ago, a Hong Kong customer visiting China would be fined, and would receive a red stamp on his return permit identifying him as a sex customer. Now, the permit is plastic and cannot receive a stamp, so a district public security bureau in Guangzhou designed a new way to punish Hong Kong customers. Once caught, the culprit must wear a signboard on his chest for one day, stating: "I use prostitutes".

Second: free operation of prostitution, which is decriminalised. Governments assist in setting up red-light zones, in which prostitutes are required to register for licences, pay tax and have regular health checks. This type of system, as operated in Germany, the Netherlands and other countries, fails to control or ensure the safety of two vulnerable groups of women: illegal immigrant prostitutes and illegally abducted foreign women forced into prostitution. In cities where there is licensed prostitution, legitimate sex workers compete with cheaper, refugee women, and helpless drug-addicted girls.

Furthermore, most prostitutes are reluctant to be licensed because nobody expects to make prostitution a lifelong career. Typically, women join the business to deal with temporary financial problems. Licensing creates a permanent record of their past. In addition, customers find unlicensed hookers more appealing because they avoid the risk of embarrassment of being seen visiting a dedicated red-light district. The licensing approach is well intentioned, but does not guarantee a complete solution.

Third: imposing management. In this case, the law admits the legality of adult prostitution and permits it within strict limits while forbidding related illegal activities such as the abduction and exploitation of women. Many countries deal with prostitution in this way, including Japan, Singapore and the United Kingdom.

From 1879 to 1932, Hong Kong had 53 years of licensed prostitution. Women were registered and paid tax. Prostitution boomed in the districts of Shek Tong Tsui, Sai Ying Pun, Wan Chai, Mong Kok and Yau Ma Tei. In the 1930s, Hong Kong had a population of less than 1,600,000, but the small client-base sex market supported 200 legal brothels with over 7,000 prostitutes. It was common practice for the over-population of prostitutes to try to physically grab passers-by for business. In 1932, the authorities issued a ban on prostitution, first on foreign prostitutes and then on locals; and three years later, licensed prostitution was ended. From that point on, Hong Kong, as a British colony, followed British practice.

British legislation paid great respect to the spirit of free trade, and as prostitution is essentially a business deal between consenting adults, it would have been inconsistent to make it illegal. As a compromise it was permitted, but subject to controls, mainly intended to keep it away from the public eye and restricted to locations known to the authorities.

Article 147, Chapter 200 of the Hong Kong legal code – 'Seducing others for indecent acts' – states that violators may receive a maximum penalty of HK$10,000 and six months' detention. Repeat offenders, or violators with criminal records, may receive a more severe punishment. In law, if a man says "What is your price?" to a female stranger on the street, he has committed the crime of 'seducing others for an indecent act'. However, customers asking prices have never been apprehended by Hong Kong police officers, while a woman on the street in an area such as Sham Shui Po might well be arrested even if seen smiling at a male passer-by.

Usually, the woman will argue that the passer-by first indicated interest, and that she did not try to bait him. The police will then summon the man as a police witness, and if he does not co-operate, the police threaten to inform his family. In court, the police will produce evidence to show the woman is of low social status, implying she would be interested in making money by any means. Naturally, the judge believes the police and their witnesses.

Living in Sham Shui Po, my friend would often be stopped by strange men who wanted to know her price. Once, she held onto such a man and called for the police to make a complaint. Rather than caution the man, the police instead warned my friend, saying: "Don't take an idle stroll on the street; you may be misunderstood."

Article 130, which is aimed at gangsters, stipulates 14 years' imprisonment as the maximum penalty for organised prostitution. Article 147 imposes a maximum punishment of HK$10,000 and six months' detention for advertising sex by way of signboards, illuminated signs and posters. To avoid prosecution, advertisements use words unrelated to sex, which has spawned a creative vocabulary open to multiple interpretations. Signboards and call-girl tabloids often use words and phrases such as 'pink glamour', 'irresistible heat', 'waiting on you', 'fleeting passion', 'cherry lips', 'daunting tits', 'exquisite relaxation', 'soothing massage', 'deep-sea diving' and 'lonely ladies'.

Articles 131 and 137 rule that people who initiate prostitution or prey on prostitutes may serve a maximum jail sentence of seven years. These articles are aimed at pimps. The high-class pimps in Hong

Kong are nightclub managers. From the legal perspective, they are bar managers who can claim to be making small talk to potential customers as a normal part of their work, and are virtually impervious to the law. However, low-level pimps cannot hide behind bar work and face tough law enforcement.

Ah Ching was a construction worker who was temporarily laid off. He cohabited with his girlfriend Ah Ling, who used to receive customers at home during the day. A plain-clothes policeman searched the house and found Ah Ching and Ah Ling in the same room. The police officer enquired about his profession and his relationship with Ah Ling. Learning he currently had no job, he was arrested and charged with procuring.

Brothel running, as described in Article 139, refers to the organised arrangement of sex deals for more than one woman or providing the facilities to do so. Premises with cashier machines or other equipment can be described as assisting prostitution, and the maximum penalty is a HK$20,000 fine and seven years' imprisonment. In Hong Kong, the most common form of legal prostitution is the '141', or one-woman brothel, which is one woman receiving customers in her apartment. If two women are found serving customers in the same apartment, it is an illegal brothel.

Sheung Shui in the New Territories was once a quiet and respectable neighbourhood. Now it is a centre of the one-woman brothel trade. The girls leave their room numbers downstairs, allowing regular customers to find them easily.

Using a tour guide agency is another way to evade law enforcement. These agencies take customers for massages to designated clock hotels, so-called because rooms are rented by the hour. During the massage, the girls may touch sensitive parts of the body and take the opportunity to offer more.

Nightclubs and karaoke bars sell drinks, entertainment and other services but have no beds. Customers may buy out the hostess for the night, and the sex deal takes place off the premises, so the law is not broken. Underground internet cafés sell a service whereby surfers may enjoy private snacks, and more, with waitresses in their computer booths.

Article 143 indicates that if leased premises are used for prostitution, violators may receive a maximum fine of HK$20,000 and seven years' imprisonment. The result is that prostitution generally takes place in old, crowded buildings with no management, facilities or regular maintenance. Landlords of these unattractive buildings are tempted to turn a blind eye, and take the easy rent while risking prosecution.

Usually it is the police who prosecute these illegal activities, with major evidence provided by the testimony of undercover officers. The limited budget of the police force prevents undercover observation of high-priced prostitutes, so the various prostitution laws usually hit the sex workers at the bottom of the pile.

In *After Suzie*, Kate Whitehead describes the undercover tricks used by Hong Kong police. Before the 1980s, a police officer would pose as a customer and have sex with the hooker. He would then reveal his identity and charge the hooker for seducing him for an indecent act. This work was popular with many police officers, who themselves became popular with prostitutes, who would offer free sex in the hope of gaining special protection. Pressured by sexually transmitted diseases, the Hong Kong police force issued a directive in 1987 to the effect that officers no longer needed to accept sexual intercourse in order to gather evidence. If officers caught a disease from their work, the police force would no longer be responsible. The directive left a grey area. Officers now ask for blowjobs.

In recent years, under the SAR government, the police have tightened their administration and have launched harsh anti-vice campaigns. Nightclub hostesses, organised tour guides and one-woman brothels can still beat the law. Street hookers are the most likely to commit the offence of 'seducing others for an indecent act'. Since they are the most vulnerable and powerless, they are the easiest to prosecute and are the hardest hit.

Busy entertainment venues can normally cover up sex deals. Massage houses and nightclubs operate on the edge of legality. To save trouble in disputes with customers, they would rather go to gangsters than to the police for settlement.

Because traditional morality condemns prostitution, women never normally entered the business voluntarily. The industry has always been dependent on gangsters to recruit economically disadvantaged but otherwise respectable women. Subsequently, they maintained control over them to keep the market supplied with workers. The illegal operating methods ensured profits and strengthened the gangsters' overall position. Until the 1980s, most Hong Kong underground sex establishments were run by gangsters who could settle any problems by bribing the police.

In the past decade, however, the Hong Kong sex industry has undergone drastic changes that have shaken the controlling power of the gangsters. Women no longer need to be coerced by gangsters. Voluntary prostitutes – including young girls, housewives, northern girls and women from Southeast Asia – have increased dramatically in number. When the supply is greater than the market demand, gangsters can no longer make a profit by coercion and their controlling power is automatically dispelled.

There is no accurate reference data about the social backgrounds of Hong Kong prostitutes, but it is certain that most come from poor families. However, with rapid economic development, there is less pressure on women to sell sex to make a living, raise funds for family medical care or pay tuition fees for younger brothers and sisters. The majority of the huge number of voluntary and part-time prostitutes are interested more in paying for a few extra luxuries, fun, and a generally enriched lifestyle.

In addition, Hong Kong is a small place with a large population and it can be difficult for women to maintain their privacy and conceal their activities, unlike on the mainland where women can make easy money under the guise of 'seeking a career in the big city', then return home to live as the good housewife.

During the Asian financial crisis, many Hong Kong women entered prostitution. Initially, their intention was to work either part-time or for a short period, but within a few months many had integrated into the business. Average-looking women pressed by money concerns found they could borrow tens of thousands of dollars from nightclub managers and madams to tide themselves over the crisis. The size of the loan determined the payback period and salary terms for a 'public relations' (PR) lady. Almost anyone willing to accept the loan terms offered by nightclub and karaoke owners can try their hand at sex work if they are desperate for money.

Alternatively, depending on the sum, a male debtor could negotiate a pimp contract or a female debtor could cut a madam deal. Once a contract is signed, the debtors are under the same pressure to pay off their loan. If the stock of females is not sufficient or not pretty enough, the pimps and madams fight for names and introductions to working girls, or even solicit girls in the street to be prostitutes.

Women choosing to enter prostitution for money do so for two reasons: they need to pay back debts for themselves or their lovers; or they are teenage beauties who can't afford their chosen lifestyle, and go to small brothel owners for a badly needed advance of HK$10,000-20,000 to be paid back through prostitution. Small brothel owners are more willing to hire under-age prostitutes, who enjoy the freedom of these unlicensed establishments until they are 18 and move on to licensed clubs.

There has been no formal research in Hong Kong into the motivation of prostitutes. Many times, I have asked the question "Why did you pick this profession?" Ah Lim dismissed the question as obsolete, telling me a better question was "Why not be a hooker?"

She continued: "Yeah, why not be a hooker? First, I'm a woman; second, I have no husband but a son to feed; third, I don't have a degree and I can't use a computer; fourth, I can sing karaoke and the hand-guessing game is easy to learn; fifth, hookers make more money in less time. So, to sum up, isn't it silly not to be a chicken? Who wants to stay home and be a dumb, boring housewife?"

Prostitutes like to claim: "I have no choice." If they were forced, they ought to be constantly plotting to break out of the prostitution prison.

The fact is, once they have decided to join the business, their affinity for the work seems to intensify while their will to seek other careers fades away. Some try to determine the logical basis for this. Since society has sympathy for miserable hookers, the most convenient excuse is that there were no other options, and so they were 'forced' from the beginning. Eventually, the notion becomes fact and they genuinely believe they are life's victims. Since they feel victimised, they believe there is no choice and that they would not be accepted elsewhere. Ironically, prostitution is a profession with a free entrance and a free exit and prostitutes are deeply drawn to this freedom. Therefore, even if offered other choices, they would still choose this freedom. Besides, Hong Kong prostitutes are superstitious and believe that they are subject to fate, so are not bound by conventional concepts of choice. As long as they can use the justification that "selling sex is just a way to make a living", ideas of quitting, changing profession or marrying out have little currency.

Young computer engineer Ah Long met a 'pure' girl in a nightclub. She bewitched him with her heartbreaking stories of what a desperate deadbeat she was, and how she had to dive into the fire just to survive. The girl saw the glowing sympathy in Ah Long's eyes and said to him, "70,000 bucks is enough. When I'm free of debt, I will quit."

It was as if she had hit his hooker-saving acupuncture point. He produced the money and the girl simply disappeared. Her madam was angry with Ah Long: "Whenever she gets money, she's gonna live fancy, and won't show up for a whole week. You made her disappear, so are you gonna pay me the debt she owes me?"

Ah Long felt disgusted by such predatory behaviour. A month later, he saw the girl in another nightclub, pure and pitiful as ever, telling the same pitiful stories, and praying for a chance to change profession. Hooker-saving heroes are as numerous as moralists who want to eradicate prostitution, but they all fail. They might as well join forces with Don Quixote.

Dodo told me that as a hooker she felt more respected than when she was a secretary. A previous boss had treated her like an office machine, while customers now treated her as a person.

Pinky quit working in a nightclub to keep house for her lover, but was dumped after two years. Feeling depressed, she swallowed a bottle and a half of poison, but was found in time and sent to hospital where her stomach was pumped. She woke up to face reality, and her first instinct was not to see her lover but to go back to whoring in the nightclub.

Kelly saved a lot of money while she was a hooker, and opened a food outlet with her boyfriend. Business was not good at the beginning, and her first impulse was not to improve the business operation but to go back to prostitution in an effort to maintain cash flow. Unfortunately, the business failed. Her boyfriend lost his savings and became desperate. Kelly just said: "No big deal. All I need is to find a new madam and hook a few customers."

# 5

# IMPORTING THE JAPANESE NIGHTCLUB

About 30 years ago, Madam Eiko introduced the Japanese-style nightclub concept to Hong Kong, and it became very influential in the world of club entertainment. The top management of nightclubs like China Town and The Big Rich would show great respect to Madam Eiko. Hong Kong gangsters never dared to start trouble or charge protection money at the nightclubs under her wing. She had lived in Hong Kong half her life and considered herself a local. She had stopped being a prostitute before coming to Hong Kong, and was viewed as a retired hooker.

Madam Eiko came from an aristocratic family in Niigata, Japan. Forty-five years ago, she was only 19 and had just graduated from high school. She worked as a clerk for half a year in a district office in Niigata but found it boring and decided to quit.

As a good lady from an aristocratic background, she received many marriage proposals, but her parents dared not agree to any of them. Eiko was a tough, blunt character fond of action. Her parents were worried that she might be sent back with a divorce certificate two weeks after the wedding. It would be too embarrassing for such a well-known family in such a small town. Eventually, her parents decided to send her to an aunt in Tokyo after she celebrated her maturity ritual, or 'adult day', at the age of 20.

While waiting for 'adult day', Eiko happened to accompany a senior family member to look for someone in the most expensive nightclub in Niigata. She was instantly drawn to the magnificent lights, glamorous costumes and noisy, happy laughter. Seeing the bar counter strewn with dirty glasses, she volunteered to help. The madam owner was rather flattered to see an aristocratic lady drop her pride to help with the dishes. She responded warmly to Eiko, telling her to come and have fun whenever she had time.

Eiko agreed, and occasionally went to help by collecting used glasses and washing dishes. She enjoyed the racy talk, carefree atmosphere, and the neverending succession of colourful characters who came to enjoy the entertainment.

Eiko was also fascinated by the madam owner, who would wear an elegant new costume every day. There was a toughness in her soft, perfectly modulated voice that complemented her expressive features. Her sense of humour entertained customers and her personality effortlessly won the girls' co-operation and customers' respect. Most of all, it was the madam's charismatic power that impressed Eiko.

The intelligent madam was gentle to everybody except her overweight husband who nagged all day long. He picked endlessly at petty faults. He was considered a total pain in the rear by girls and customers alike. The madam would greet customers with grace, cajole hostesses into a good mood when sending them out to customers; and then suddenly, she could shower biting abuse on her husband, without turning a hair. In a split second, her expression could change from one extreme to another.

Between one moment and the next, beauty, graceful dignity, purity, feminine serenity and power were all on display on the madam's face. How could this mortal world contain such a beautiful woman, living such an intoxicating life? Eiko knew then that she could never live as a traditional wife. The radiant glamour of the madam had shown her an alternative.

Eiko rushed to Tokyo immediately after her maturity ritual. In spite of her family's opposition, she became a drinking companion in a small bar in Ginza. Very quickly, a high-class nightclub tempted her away with double the salary. Two years later, the most famous nightclub in Ginza approached her with an offer of even more money. Later, she started working as a prostitute and became the mistress of three rich men. When she had learned enough about nightclub operation and built up a group of regular patrons, she asked her lovers to help her open a club in Akasaka.

As she approached 30, Eiko had become experienced in the nightclub business and married another shrewd nightclub owner. Their own nightclub, however, went into bankruptcy at the time a friend wanted to give away his Japanese-style bar in Hong Kong. Eiko accepted the offer and came to Hong Kong with her husband. They turned the bar into a Ginza-style operation and it became the first Japanese nightclub in Hong Kong.

The entertainment business is all about public relations. Although following precise rules and rituals, the Ginza-style operation was flexible enough to cater successfully to various customers' needs.

Hong Kong locals came to Eiko to learn her management style, which was adapted for use in large local nightclubs like China City, Tonnochy and Club Bboss.

Eiko said: "It may seem silly that I decided to join the profession out of envy of the madam owner in Niigata, but Japan didn't offer women many opportunities to rebel against its patriarchal regime. After all, I'm an aristocrat, so I have to be the best no matter what I do. Perhaps meeting that madam owner and eventually teaching the Japanese nightclub style in Hong Kong was my fate."

# 6

# LAU KEIKEI

"Lau Keikei" is an alias the interview subject was keen for me to use, because it contains the Chinese character for "wood". During our two hours together her sensitivity and eloquence quickly drew me into her life story. It is my policy not to pay interview fees, so that the subjects are discouraged from elaborating their stories. Indeed, that was our initial understanding. However, after hearing her full account, I felt humbled and the payment of a fee seemed the least I could do.

It was Lau Keikei's large, violet eyes that first caught my attention – hollow eyes that had seen their share of misery. Then there were her vain efforts to cover her mouth to hide the fact she had no front teeth. On several occasions she bragged: "I was a hostess in The Capital of Flowers club when I was young. Back then, we learned how to make-up, how to dance, how to act gracefully, how to keep regular customers entertained with good conversation. Not like the girls today; shit, all they know is how to fuck."

One night, I returned to a side lane off Temple Street, a regular pitch for seven or eight street girls. There was a chill in the air and I was bringing some old clothes for the girls, who were happy to try them on except for Lau Keikei. She thought the clothes were not sexy enough, so she walked away.

A little boy was playing nearby on the pavement with a model car. He was pushing it to see how far it would run on its own. The toy car bumped into a lamppost, flipped over, then rolled out into the middle of the road. The boy ran into the road just as a large lorry approached.

Keikei exclaimed: "Watch out, kid!" She dropped the cigarette she had just lit, dashed out in front of the lorry and grabbed the little boy. It was then that his mother appeared; without a word she roughly snatched the boy away, half turning her back towards Keikei, who almost lost her balance and fell over. She dragged her son away with one hand over her nose, as if she was rescuing him from something rotten.

"What a rude woman!" I said, quite angry at the woman's behaviour.

"You do ask for trouble!" said one of the other girls trying on clothes. "I may have fucked her husband," said Keikei, as she picked up her cigarette and took a drag as if nothing had happened. "She still had no right to treat you like shit," said the other girl. I found Keikei's calm response strangely irritating.

"I have fucked plenty. I really might have done her husband." She continued to smoke, reflecting on the possibility.

Inaccurately applied lipstick and eyeliner did nothing to conceal a legacy of tired, waxen skin from 25 tough years of prostitution and drugs. Untidy dress, greasy hair, and the puffiness of an unfit middle-aged body seemed in keeping with the shabby street; yet, just a moment ago, this person had showed an unexpected agility and willingness to save an unknown child.

In the year of Hong Kong's return to Chinese sovereignty, the media headlines made a posthumous celebrity of Lee Ying Kwong, who had sacrificed his life trying to save a child struggling in the currents of an overflowing river. There was a collection in order to help the hero's family deal with its loss of income. When two Mrs Lees came forward for the money, there was an abrupt halt to the adulation of the new hero. Several TV stations were determined to find a sexual angle in the heated debate of whether or not Mr Lee should be crowned a hero. In the end, Hong Kong citizens forgave Lee Ying Kwong for the dishonesty in his private life, which does not necessarily cause any logical conflict with the noble act of his sacrifice. The general public was willing to give his memory an honourable funeral.

If Lau Keikei had been crushed by the lorry while saving the child, would she have received the same honour? It's most unlikely. Although the selfless nature of the act is comparable, half of Hong Kong's population are 'good women', and the other half would not dare to make outspoken remarks in support of a street hooker.

A fortune-teller told a mother that her newborn daughter would put the family in debt and cause trouble. In that same year, the father was wounded at work. He was unable to earn a penny during several months of sick leave. Neither could the family afford medication for a grandfather on his deathbed. These events served only to convince the mother and grandmother of the accuracy of the fortune-teller's prediction.

All Lau Keikei can remember of her childhood is a distant, disciplinarian mother and a stone-hearted grandmother who treated her younger brother and sister quite differently, with love and devotion. Keikei thought she was not good enough in some way, so to win her mother's approval she decided to busy herself with housework. This was when she was five years old, and from that time she effectively became the family maid. When she was 12, she passed the entrance exam for a church school, but her mother said: "You should earn some family income to help your sisters and brothers at school."

She found work in a factory and a young man there pursued her constantly. He was so spellbound that he decided he could not live a single day without her. This unstinting love and attention so compensated for her loveless childhood that she did not mind her new boyfriend was a drug dealer. Later, he offered a considerable dowry to her parents, which was accepted.

After they married, her husband was often beaten up for not paying his debts. When the couple could take the violence no longer, they decided to pay off the debts by letting Keikei work in a nightclub as a hostess.

At the beginning, Keikei only made money from her time working in the club, which wasn't enough to clear the debt. The madam then talked her into sleeping with customers, taking them to Kowloon Tong, where there are many 'love hotels'.

After overcoming her initial reluctance and becoming a regular visitor to Kowloon Tong, she finally earned enough to settle her husband's debt. The experience had taught her how to attract customers and how to encourage them to spend freely. She had mastered the trick of how to handle men. This gave her a confidence she never knew before and it made her want to carry on with the business.

From her years of experience, she knew from the moment she answered Mr Chan's call that he was a naturally sympathetic and charitable man. She decided not to rush to a sex deal and rejected several offers, and although she finally went to Kowloon Tong with him, she remained coy. There was only mild foreplay and no lovemaking.

When they finally did make love, she refused to accept payment. Mr Chan was so flattered that he told her to quit. She made up a story that she owed her company HK$100,000 and had to keep working. Mr Chan immediately gave her the money. This generosity reminded her of how her husband used to be. She was genuinely touched and accepted her feelings for him.

She had no reason to go on working, so she dined with Mr Chan every day. He respected her and did not touch her. She knew he wanted to take her in and look after her. She was grateful and wanted to have a real romance with him, sacrificing the fun she had at the nightclub. Unfortunately, his meek style left her feeling no passion at all. When Mr Chan eventually raised the issue of marriage, she knew she was not ready to be a dutiful housewife and felt unworthy of this kind of love. But she also knew she may never again have such an opportunity for a good, normal life, and decided to leave her drug-dealer husband.

Fearing her husband's violence, she packed up when he was not at home, and though it had gone well, just as she was about to leave she received a blow to the head from a baseball bat that knocked her out cold. When she awoke, she found herself tied to the bed with her husband interrogating her endlessly about her lover. He injected her with heroin over a period of ten days to make sure she was truly addicted, and then released her.

For Mr Chan's safety, she could not go back to The Capital of Flowers nightclub. Keikei genuinely did care about him, and bemoaned: "Just one fuck cost him that much; even if he filled my pussy with diamonds I would not let him get beaten for his generosity."

Keikei started work in the Oriental Palace nightclub. Now she was drug-addicted, she had no interest in sex and no longer took pleasure in hunting men. Her husband watched her like a hawk. He controlled her bank account and waited for her to finish working every night to take a cut of her money.

She found it impossible to hold down the job at the Oriental Palace and started to work hotel lobbies and then the waiting rooms of gambling dens. She went from handjob and blowjob brothels to a one-woman brothel, and ended up as a street hooker. She just went through the motions with her customers; her mind was elsewhere, preoccupied with how to get a little more love from her husband. She tried so hard to look after him and win him back from other women that she had no energy to look after herself. No longer feeling either, she gave up trying to distinguish between love and hate. Heroin was now the only thing that allowed her to feel anything at all. It had ruined her health and was rotting her body from the inside out. She had begun to lose teeth at the age of 30, and within five years, all her front teeth were gone.

In recent years, the dead bodies of addicted street hookers have been found in public rest rooms, by the roadside, and in piles of garbage. Keikei saw this as her own destiny. Dying in this way ensures that no family will come forward to claim the body.

She wanted to see her mother again. To gain her favour, she had been paying HK$1,000 a month into her mother's bank account, no matter how poor or downcast she was. After a year, she felt she had paved the way to meet her mother, but realised how bad she would look without a full set of teeth.

As an outcast from the family, she was extremely sensitive and wary when talking about her mother. She recalled their last meeting at her sister's wedding.

When Keikei was married, her mother demanded a huge dowry. This forced her husband to take out a number of loans to cover the cost of both the dowry and the wedding ceremony. Despite benefiting from the handsome dowry, her mother came to the wedding empty-handed. She did not even bother to make a token attempt at giving the customary gift of jewellery. The bride and groom were so embarrassed that they had to borrow jewellery on the spot to save face. With tears in her heart, she had to tell white lies to the guests, saying "Mother gave me this jewellery" while displaying the borrowed items for inspection.

Being superstitious, her husband believed that her mother avoided blessing them with gifts in order to place a curse on their marriage. Keikei found herself in the position of making up a million excuses for her mother.

The next year, Keikei's sister was married. Their mother lavished gifts of jewellery on the bride. Keikei's psychological defences completely broke down at the wedding, not from envy of her sister's jewellery, but because she could no longer make excuses for her mother. While talking about her sister's wedding, tears welled in her worldly eyes which now looked so fragile and childlike.

For years, Keikei took three fixes of heroin every day. She continued picking up a few customers, but did not think about what she was doing, what she wanted to do, what she should do, or what she could do. She had no fear of dying on the street, but she did want to see her mother. Her sister and brother sympathised with her, and her mother gradually realised her superstition and coldness had ruined Keikei's life. Even so, a meeting was going to be very difficult after years of separation. Keikei felt that it should be a very solemn and significant occasion, for which she needed good dentures.

Keikei developed a plan. Firstly, she would go to a rehabilitation clinic to rid herself of drug addiction. If her mother accepted her, she would then find work as a waitress or dishwasher, and take her mother to teahouses during festivals and holidays. This project required HK$50,000. The dentures alone would cost HK$20,000, and to survive cold turkey would cost a further HK$30,000. She tried twice to give up the drug habit, but her savings ran out during the rehabilitation period, before she could get a new job. She had to pick up the old profession again, and went back to heroin.

During field research in Sham Shui Po, as a volunteer social worker with Blue Bird (the Catholic NGO concerned with the welfare of sex workers), I often came across another big-eyed girl who was besotted with her boyfriend. Sister Ai told me that Big Eyes was with Keikei's ex-husband.

Once, Big Eyes took out two ID cards and asked me: "Madam, I want to marry him inside the prison. We can apply for public housing if we are legitimately married, so when he's out, we'll have a place to live. Could you help me out with the procedures?" It looked as if Big Eyes loved the man just as much as Lau Keikei had. To me, the man in the picture on the ID card looked like a stereotypical gangster. A second look at the ID card rooted me to the spot; the man's name was Lau Kei.

My heart cried out: Lau Keikei, you are still in love with the man who destroyed your life. After all he has done, you keep his name. You have told me all about the tragedies in your life, but not who you really are.

Lau Keikei may have blamed herself for falling for the wrong man, but to prove fate wrong, she had made up her mind to love Lau Kei utterly and forever.

At 38 years old, Lau Keikei has no money, no family, no dignity, not even a complete face, and no strength to believe that she is a person worth loving. She really has nothing. But I know that if she could buy herself a 'mouth-gate' (her word), it would be a great victory in her own small world. She would feel stronger, love herself a little more, and feel able to see her mother.

*Postscript*

Blue Bird and I wrote a fundraising prospectus on behalf of Lau Keikei, to help her rehabilitation. We delivered the prospectus to several charity organisations. A well-known Hong Kong philanthropist donated HK$20,000 to Blue Bird, giving a specific instruction that it be used for Lau Keikei's dentures.

With her new teeth, Lau Keikei managed to quit the street for six months, but then fell back into prostitution and drugs. Two years later, I met Lau Keikei and asked if she had seen her mother. She pretended that she didn't understand what I was talking about, and tried to avoid talking to me.

Last year, teachers and students of sociology from Hong Kong Polytechnic University asked for Lau Keikei's contact details for their research. Keikei thanked me for the introduction, and doubled her interview charge. She also gave consent for a video record; filming her back would double the interview charge again, while filming her face would be triple. The researchers chose the rear view.

This time, her name was Wen Wen instead of Lau Keikei, and her life story was wonderfully told, but it was completely different to the version given to me. The details varied throughout, but the themes remained the same, stressing that she was a good person forced to deteriorate and become a prostitute; despite adversity she had kept her love alive, and had been generous to friends.

She included some sleazy material to cater to the prurient interests of the interviewers, saying that she once met a pervert who asked to drink her urine. At first I felt cheated and angry, but then I was overwhelmed by sadness. It was very hard to hold back my tears until the end of her fabrication.

Did Lau Keikei ever tell me a single word of the truth? Which version was closer to her real life? Had she faked her tears when telling me about her sister's wedding?

Maybe it's too harsh to label her a phoney. The story of Lau Keikei reveals three paradoxical truths.

Although lacking the benefit of a basic education, she had enough wit to realise what kind of stories would satisfy intellectuals and academics. Although a member of the most disadvantaged group, at the very bottom of the social ladder, she had enough guile to convince me, and then a philanthropist, to raise money for her dentures. And although her income from sex work could not cover her basic necessities, her story holds value in the media and in areas of academic research.

# 7

## WHAT'S ON THE MENU?

It seems that approximately two-thirds of punters are primarily interested in sexual pleasure, while 16% just want a change of face, and presumably body. The remainder claim to want to let someone else do the work for a change, paying the prostitute to make all the moves; so found Professor Shan Naiguang of the Beijing Academy of Social Science during his research. Professor Shan also found demand was moving away from basic sexual intercourse to alternative practices.

Traditionally, in the absence of any other source of information about sex techniques, Chinese prostitutes have studied classic pornographic literature. The time-honoured approach is to adopt the style of the coquette. The secret lies in developing a come-hither look, hinting at sexual possibilities. There is an old saying along the lines of "One can be overcome by just a look". The art of suggestion, then, is supposedly all it takes.

Once, during fieldwork in Sham Shui Po, I witnessed a plain-looking girl give a coy look to a young man bargaining with her colleagues. The coy look sealed the deal: he left the group and approached the plain girl who softly said, "This way". She led him, hips swaying, key dangling from her finger, to her room.

The prostitutes I know all think coquetry is indeed a good trick to learn. It has worked for thousands of years by effectively exploiting the male tendency to judge sexual attractiveness quickly and visually. However, this trick is losing its audience. Hong Kong prostitutes now find they will likely end up penniless, and kicked out of the whore house, if they rely simply on making themselves available as passive receptacles after a few flutters of the eyelashes.

When my parents were young, the same bar of soap would be used for washing clothes, hair, face, feet, and bathing. Nowadays, if the supermarket sold only one brand of soap, it would be evidence of a poor economy and high unemployment. To appease the consumer vanity that comes with affluence, manufacturers have learnt the appeal of offering choice. The basic ingredients may be similar, but they can be packaged as hair shampoo, shower gel, washing up liquid, laundry detergent, floor cleaner and so on. Hair products are further divided to suit greasy, normal or dry hair; they offer tangle resistance, UV protection, and treatments for dandruff, grey hair, split ends and falling hair. Choice becomes an expected part of consumerism. The consumer tendency to expect choice spreads to all commodities, including entertainment and sex.

Sex in the mass media takes the form of endless variations of erotic images, pornographic movies, magazines and novels, sex toys, live performances, internet sex and phone sex. Even cocktails have joke names like 'sex on the beach' and 'screaming orgasm'. This provides employment and profits for filmmakers, newspapers, photographers, printers, manufacturers of sex toys, prostitutes, novelists, and the list goes on. Vested interests are constantly under pressure to develop and present new variations, to excite further demand and new audiences.

It was inevitable that sex comprising nothing more than a flirty look and an uninspired missionary interlude, with maybe a few standard variations, was one day going to lose its attraction among an increasingly aware, affluent and curious customer base.

Commercial sex, forever craving new fantasies, changes consumers' sexual tastes, and recruits otherwise conventional, straight, ordinary men and women into the multifaceted marketplace. Japanese pornographers have had a distinctive approach. They tend to separate sexual joy from the sexual organs. To pander to the Japanese male psyche, there is little if any attempt to suggest the humanity of the participants.

Japanese pornography tends to include the following themes:

- Originally noble characters are turned into worthless sluts who find their real joy only when they are bullied and debased.

- Couples and lovers are replaced with perverted or bestial relationships including such combinations as teacher and student, nurse and patient, housewife and postman, daughter and school friend, humans and various creatures such as dogs and farm animals, and variations of incest.

- Foreplay leads to consummation in a series of public places and situations.

- Objectification of the human body is achieved by the frequent use of plastic toys and sundry apparatus.

All these aspects have one thing in common: the tendency to portray embarrassing fantasies, often associated with shame and humiliation.

Hong Kong men also seem to have a need for a type of virtual sex. It has been observed that Hong Kong women, although economically independent, hold conservative attitudes towards sex compared to other urban women in Taiwan and mainland China. Three structural factors seem to explain this conservatism.

Firstly, primary and secondary education in Hong Kong is predominantly provided by Christian and Catholic schools, as well as a number of Buddhist schools. School leavers from such institutions will likely be further influenced by a family background imbued with Confucian values, which leads to a mindset concerning sex built on dual ideological rigidity. Traditional Taoist beliefs include notions of sex for procreation only, with little emphasis on pleasure. Indeed, Taoism teaches men to save their vital essences to retain their strength and vigour. These factors tend to produce sexually naive young men and women with little more than token sexual experience before marriage, which explains many of the subsequent behaviour patterns.

Secondly, most young people live with their families in crowded apartments and have few opportunities to pursue sexual freedom.

Thirdly, Hong Kong women are faced with a harshly competitive marketplace for men because Hong Kong men have abundant choices when seeking lovers, wives, mistresses and prostitutes in mainland China or other less-developed areas.

Hong Kong women tend to seek emotional security in serious relationships, and make use of traditional gender values to cultivate feelings of responsibility in men. In return, women are expected to behave in an inward, sexually innocent and passive manner.

Hong Kong men find little sexual release in dealing with these cold, passionless angels. The answer is Japanese-made pornography, which they inform with their own repressed, non-verbalised desires. This allows them to construct a composite woman who is an angel in social circumstances but turns into a sex-hungry whore in bed when subjected to the man's sexual skills. The same conservatism that produces cold angels also produces sexually ignorant and inept men. Many Hong Kong wives find sex uninteresting and exhausting because everything they know is learnt from their husbands.

The husbands reap what they sow. Putting little effort into communicating with their wives in order to develop satisfying sex, they become frustrated and seek compensation in commercial sex where they can buy a seemingly satisfactory response apparently lacking in their wives.

*Apple Daily* and *Oriental Daily* reported that a Japanese pornographic film company once sent Grade Four (hard-core) film stars and Japanese strippers to Mong Kok in Hong Kong, to promote their films to a dedicated audience. The venue was packed and the anonymous strippers drew almost as much adulation as would an established Hollywood movie star.

Hong Kong men find particular solace in Japanese porn that depicts quite ordinary males displaying typically modest endowments and women who appear to show only reluctant or passive compliance.

This preference is confirmed by market stall vendors, who report that Japanese pornographic DVDs enjoy huge sales, not only because of their production quality but also because of their stylised approach and novel, fashionable sexual practices. Despite the plot and language, most Japanese movies reinforce the same message: innocent, passive girls enjoy aggressive sex with savage men and are compliant in causing their own pain and humiliation.

Men watch sex movies at home only for the purpose of sexual pleasure, and usually for masturbation. Regular buyers of Japanese discs are normally male professionals between 35 and 50, maybe married, with a mortgage, living a stereotypical life. These men include husbands who make concessions to wives, single men with lovers to please, men with senior female colleagues, men who submit to female bosses, and men who may be humiliated by female customers, or even ridiculed by female clients. Watching pornographic movies with the theme of humiliating women is virtual revenge. However, having seen new ideas in these movies, how do these men achieve the actual experience? It would be unthinkable for them to approach their cold-angel wives or lovers.

The Hong Kong media have experienced a revolution in the promotion of sex information. During the last ten years, sex magazines such as *Salty Spongy Square, Wild Nights, Call Girl Directory, Sex Convenience Store* and *Pimp Guide* have flourished. Newspapers now hire professional pimps to edit columns giving readers information about sex establishments and their girls, their prices and sex tricks. One effect has been mushrooming interest in sexual techniques such as 'three heavens of ice and fire', 'oil-soaked sparrow', 'dragon drill', 'dragon spitting pearls', 'mouth explosion', 'wet blow', 'face bang', SM, and others.

Magazines, movies, erotic novels, sex toys, sexy celebrity women and an increasing use of nude photography create a push-pull effect. The porn industry is ever-inventive and its sex workers must try ever harder to meet the hunger for new sensations.

Perhaps conventional prostitutes survived on the art of coquetry for generations, but these days, those slow to learn and adapt will be left behind. The new professionals must cater to this hunger for novelty and fantasy.

The appetite for pornography has undoubtedly increased among Hong Kong men. A survey by the Chinese University of Hong Kong's Sociology Department indicates that 275,000 new customers emerged during the economic downturn in the second half of 2002.

There is a structural mismatch between greater demand for fantasy fulfilment by Hong Kong men, and the generally conservative attitudes of Hong Kong women, which are a matter of record. If wives and lovers, for various reasons, are unapproachable, prostitutes are an available supply to meet the demand.

At one time just spreading their legs was sufficient, but to stay in business today, prostitutes must offer a set of five or seven 'flavours', similar in principle to a set menu in a restaurant, based on a fixed price for a set number of courses. Enterprising girls will make the effort to be more inventive and offer further variations, including specialising in the more difficult techniques.

The basic five-flavour set includes: 1) shower with the customer, 2) oral sex with mouthwash, 3) rimming, 4) toe licking, and 5) vaginal intercourse. The seven-flavour set would include two extra tricks, such as a particular form of aggressive anal sex in which the customer holds the girl down by the back of her neck to restrict her movements. The restraint feature is critical as it increases the client's satisfaction by emphasising the girl's vulnerability and humiliation.

Another popular practice is 'three heavens of ice and fire', which involves oral sex with alternating mouthfuls of hot tea, ice cubes and mouthwash. The three 'heavens' are hot, cold and astringent.

Being prepared to offer a 'dragon drill' on the five- and seven-flavour menus is a must for all nightclub workers. It is a version of analingus in which the critical sensation is to feel the girl's active tongue being pushed as far as possible into the anus.

Outside nightclubs, many customers are willing to pay an extra HK$3,000 to receive 'dragon drill' from professional massage girls in private clubs. It is understood that for Hong Kong men, knowing that the girl is *un*willing to perform 'dragon drill' makes it a particularly special treat.

At the lower end of the sex market, it is common practice that additional payment is demanded for any tricks other than regular sex. If a client goes to a cheap hooker for the five- or seven-flavour set, each course is charged separately, which can be expensive. It is for this reason that customers would rather go to a nightclub girl and ask directly if she will do the tricks for an inclusive price.

Refusal means no business. Previously, nightclub customers did not dare to request special tricks, and if they did, they were usually met with a flat refusal. But today, Hong Kong nightclubs suffer greatly from competition from nightclubs within easy travelling distance in mainland China. To survive, high class Hong Kong prostitutes have to offer the five- or seven-flavour sets, and even more demanding sex tricks.

Ah Choi has been a hostess in a nightclub for six years. She said: "To do the five or seven flavours is a daily routine for us, and I still haven't got used to it after all these years. Not because I hate my profession, but because these flavour sets are just not for humans."

Melissa, a nightclub mama-san, told me: "Customers today bring in sex magazines like a menu, telling me they want this, they want that. So I tell the girls: If you don't want to do it, there are others who will. Under these circumstances, how can the girls refuse anal sex, oral sex or group sex? They will take on almost anything, or they have no business. Customers seem addicted to the novel tricks, trying out one after another. The girls have to agree, to keep customers hooked. The market is seeing new stuff at an amazing speed. Nevertheless, prostitutes are still just flesh and blood, so how can they keep going when asked all these requests? The girls begin to shake the minute they punch in for work; they have no idea what kind of strange requests customers will make during the long night ahead."

Melissa complained: "This 'sex fad' culture is such a sin. Customers used to flirt with the girls, and this would develop into friendship when they were really in the mood. Customers today all seem to have been genetically modified overnight; they come just to pay for various sex games. The girls have been modified as well. They used to learn to dance, to communicate, to dress up, to study men's mentality; they were subtle and warm-hearted; even knowledgeable about current events. In order to make conversation, they'd ask a financier about the Hang Seng Index, or ask a developer for advice about property. Prostitutes today have all become sex slaves. Numb like wooden chickens, they just sit there, eating and drinking at the customer's expense with no manners at all. They don't even bother to enquire about how the gentleman would like to be addressed, whether or not they should use his family name. Instead, they simply push the customers to buy them out of the club. How can the customers respect these silly chickens? It's not surprising they just treat them like boring sex toys. The girls ask for it."

Dely, another mama-san, had no complaints about the changing fashions in sex. Her advice is to face the reality with gusto, instead of being nostalgic for the way things used to be. She warns her girls: "Try to keep your dignity and you'll starve."

Every day she coaches her girls patiently: "Coquetry is something for celebrity women, models, for stars to flirt with rich brats. Focused sex has become our speciality. Every profession specialises. Nightclub girls are expensive sex workers, and their selling point is sex novelty. So, to attract customers, they must master many sex tricks. A simple fuck, and a few moans to make the client feel good, is no longer enough, so everybody practises *chi kung* and learns how to contract their vaginal muscles."

Some of the mama-sans were kind enough to let me sit in the waiting rooms of their nightclubs so I could chat with the girls. When I asked them who the most troublesome customers were, they nearly always gave the same answers: flagellators, those who can't get it up, and those who can't come.

Skinny Helen said: "I don't mind 'three heavens of ice and fire', except for the limp noodles. No matter if I give beer, or I give XO, I just can't squeeze a single drop out of it. If not for the money, I'd rather not suck this, suck that every day."

When asked who the best customers are, they have different answers.

19-year-old Pinky said: "My best customer gets hard the second he walks into the room, and I don't need to give him a blow job. But some customers take aphrodisiacs or Viagra, so if you don't blow them, they'll bang you for ages, it really knocks you out."

Winnie said: "My favourite one asks me to play dead. He only comes making love to dead people. Now that's easy, I just shut my eyes for a few minutes, then I get the money. But there are so few like that."

40-year-old Margaret said she didn't mind impotent customers: "It's good if it's not hard, then I can suggest some ideas to help, and charge him more."

Ah Yan once met a customer she thought was decent, but he tied her up as soon as they were alone together. Ah Yan was petrified, begging him not to kill her. After a while, the customer told her that it was a joke, and he paid her well after releasing her. Ah Yan thought it was a good deal, and put that customer on the VIP list. When he came again, the girls fought for him and it was Ah Sum that he bought out. She made no extra money because she was mentally prepared, and the customer thought she wasn't frightened enough. Ah Sum was angry: "Was I in a horror movie? He should go to a cinema school. I just fuck, and I'm good at it!"

Ah Ngo was in a clock hotel (rented by the hour) when suddenly the customer whipped her twice on her buttocks, and later paid her HK$500. When she returned to the club, she complained: "500 bucks to lash my ass, no way! No more freaks for me." However, when he returned, she needed money badly, so she offered him the same deal.

Zhang Wuji used many women but he said he never beat or humiliated a hostess. He just wanted to try new sex games. "Prostitution is a way to taste new dishes, which is the purpose of the sex treat. Otherwise, why not go home for family meals?"

Another popular service is called the 'outdoor bang'. Instead of using a clock hotel, customers like to drive to a not-so-remote street corner and have sex in the car, demanding the girl screams loudly to give the thrill of the risk of discovery. Others prefer the romance of a park environment, so they have sex with the girls outside, against the car, surrounded by trees and falling leaves. Given the choice, some hostesses would rather take a whipping, because they fear being seen outside in public. In addition, they don't want the marks left by mosquito bites over their arms and legs, which puts off customers and is bad for business.

Some customers like to go Dutch. Two men each buy out a girl and take them to the same room for the night. They take turns to have both vaginal and anal sex with both girls. Each man pays just one girl.

A self-proclaimed beauty from Beijing, who would charge top dollar for her services, once met a very decent customer who asked her to kneel down naked and worship his not-so-decent penis like praying to an idol in a temple. She had to assume a meek and subservient role, or the customer would refuse to pay.

Ah Kuen had been working for many years and wasn't a big name even when she was young and pretty. However, each time she became pregnant, she was able to attract a lot of her regular customers and new clients who were willing to pay extra to suckle her milk. For the sake of money, Ah Kuen would carry on this business until she was eight months pregnant and very obviously with child.

Man-man told me that 'oil-soaked sparrow' is a tough trick. It means the girl has to be patient and willing to coax and cajole a tiny penis. Only when the customer ejaculates is the sparrow 'oil-soaked'.

Some customers go to Ah Fung with sex toys, carrots, cucumbers and much more. Ah Fung takes this on, charging an additional HK$100. Her worst customers insert various candy bars and desserts, take them out and ask her to eat them, and be happy while doing so.

Chinese customers with traditional tastes like to visit pitiful prostitutes. To play the miserable wretch is the stock-in-trade of the conventional coquette prostitute. First, the customer listens to her sad story, then makes a show of pity and sympathy, which gives him huge satisfaction as it flatters his position of relative power and ability to relieve her suffering. After the deal, the girl shows due gratitude, and the customer enjoys his role as benefactor.

Two hostesses working under mama-san Stella could not adapt to changing tastes. They would follow the traditional pattern of recounting their pitiful history to their customers, who were not interested and would complain to Stella. The night after I first met Stella, I saw her yelling at the two 'pitiful' hostesses: "Now the economy is sluggish, everybody is suffering for real, not like the make-believe stories you two sick chickens tell customers. If you keep on playing the pitiful wretch, telling your sad stories, you can quit this work and start begging!"

The two girls didn't feel too bad after being scolded. They even asked with a smile: "If we don't play the pitiful wretch, what role should we play?" Stella hopped onto the low table in the waiting room and announced, "Now the economy is heading downhill, every man needs to be cheered up, so all you girls work your asses off and play the sex-crazed monster or the demanding bitchy slut!"

Mary, another mama-san, didn't agree with Stella. She was worried that the inexperienced girls would blow it by overacting the sexy slut. She stressed: "When you play the sexy bitch, you should try not to seem too experienced; men don't like over-experienced sluts."

One hostess retorted: "We only do the five and seven flavours, what does it matter if we just add two more? If you keep telling us to play this and play that, don't be mad if we switch to another mama-san."

Mary was quite upset but dared not offend her hostesses. She carefully brought up the matter of customers' complaints, one of which was that a girl had begun to scream immediately after lying down: "Fuck me hard, screw my pussy", and the customer came in just a few seconds. He was not very happy.

For many customers, the best part is picking the hostess. In Hong Kong, especially in high-class nightclubs, replacing the suggested girl has been unpopular because it would hurt the girl's self-esteem, having a negative impact on business. The success of nightclubs in nearby Shenzhen has attracted many men from Hong Kong because the girls there will line up to be chosen. The Hong Kong sex industry understands this psychology perfectly well and a low-class nightclub on Portland Street offered a variation of offering multiple replacements. A customer could pick from a line-up of five girls and replace them all if not satisfied; he could then pick from another five and replace all of them again, and so on.

This became extremely popular and other nightclubs simply had to follow suit. This service required the establishments to employ large numbers of northern girls from the mainland, because the more expensive Hong Kong prostitutes would not agree to the line-ups. According to a local news report in October 2003, a customer was beaten to death after multiple replacing. This led to the end of the practice in the Hong Kong sex market.

To gain a competitive edge, a brothel in Jordan promoted a new deal: HK$100/4Q, meaning that if a customer could come four times within an hour, he would be charged only HK$100 for everything. Even though the most virile man would have difficulty achieving four orgasms an hour, the promotion still attracted a long queue from the front door and out onto the pavement. Since the hopeful customers generally failed to score a '4', and accepted other services such as a shower, erotic massage and oral sex, they typically ended up paying at least HK$350.

Alternative sex practised in Hong Kong is not necessarily sado-masochistic, and can be more psychologically driven, from the exercise of power to subtly destroying the sex worker's dignity.

I asked the girls what they disliked most about their work and 90% of them said that they could accept virtually anything – except not being paid afterwards or not being paid enough. This is seen as more humiliating than the most weird of their clients' requests. If not supported by a mama-san or protected by an organised club environment, they would need to pay regular protection money to boyfriends or pimps to prevent this insult. Anyone who dares not to pay would likely receive a severe beating, not only to retrieve the money, but more significantly to save the dignity of the sex worker.

Ada was too shy to ask directly for payment after her first deal. The customer took advantage by not raising the matter and simply sent her away. Ada felt as depressed as if she had been raped, regretting even more that it had happened after she had made the trip to visit the client. She had sold her body and not been paid. The more she thought about it, the angrier she became. She felt she would rather be dead.

Her mama-san later found out what happened. Without a word, she paid Ada herself and comforted her. She had the customer found and demanded he return the money and apologise to Ada. The mama-san severely upbraided the customer, stressing that prostitution without payment is a callous act that strips the girl of her dignity.

Prostitution activists view the pursuit of increased variety in sex as part of the phenomenon of sexual liberation, and presumably sexual pleasure. If alternative practices resulting from sexual liberation are truly pleasurable, then why can Hong Kong men not find willing lovers to perform them? Why must they resort to sex workers to lick their anuses and toes, supply human milk, and provide orifices for vegetables and candy bars, in order to express their newly found liberation?

In the absence of any imminent social or sexual revolution, Hong Kong women seem to have only two choices: either force themselves to accept special requests from their husbands and boyfriends, or accept that their husbands and boyfriends will search for fun elsewhere. Hong Kong prostitutes also have two choices: either refuse to accept requests for alternative sex, or actively take part and even design new variations to win over, and keep, customers.

# 8

## NORTHERN GIRLS

Of the estimated global population of peasants of 2.3 billion, China has 0.9 billion or 40%. The book *Investigation of Chinese Peasants* by Chen Guidi and Chun Tao is a work of investigative journalism that was officially banned in China, because it openly points out that economic reform in the post-Mao era has created powerful local oligarchies in rural areas which have worsened peasants' livelihoods.

Previously, the deep-rooted parochial mindset of Chinese peasantry made it unthinkable for people to leave their land and village, but now, peasants swarm to the cities and are prepared to accept tremendous hardship and prejudice to achieve the financial benefits of finding better-paid work. Traditionally, peasant women have been commoditised as household labourers, prostitutes, slaves, servants, wives and concubines. These practices had been strictly controlled in Mao's China, but soon after his regime ended, these 'traditions' were actually reinforced by economic reform as market-driven urban areas absorbed the endless supply of rural female labour, fertility and sexuality. With the relaxation of state control in post-Mao China, many young peasant girls began to leave their villages to sell their sexuality in cities.

At a Hong Kong seminar on prostitution in China, Professor Shan of the Beijing Academy of Social Science pointed out that very few mainland prostitutes were forced into the profession. Only 1.3% could be considered as pressurised, e.g. coming from families desperate for money, coaxed to believe in the supposedly high potential income or lured by girls from the same village into prostitution in cities. The huge income discrepancy between rural and urban workers means that a single country girl can easily make a whole family's annual income through prostitution. This has drastically increased the number of mainland prostitutes working without any coercion by gangsters.

Due to the strict official ban on prostitution, it is necessary to operate surreptitiously, as part of a black economy. Chinese authorities have no clear idea of the total number of girls or their social impact. Police data gives a clear picture of the dramatic relative increase of prostitution, but not the overall number of girls involved.

Before the economic reforms, the Guangzhou Public Security Bureau would arrest only a few prostitutes each year. By the end of the 1970s, the annual arrest total was 39 but by the end of the 1980s the annual number had risen to 5,000. In 1998, over 10,000 prostitutes were arrested. There is no information as to how many escaped the police. Prostitutes are shrewd enough to dodge the police in places where prostitution has been established for a long time. Among the arrests made by the Guangzhou Public Security Bureau, 10% were rural and illiterate, 25% had finished elementary school, 50% had a junior high education, approximately 14% had graduated from senior high school, and only 1% were college graduates.

Typically, unmarried rural girls of 18 to 29 years old would tell their families they were seeking jobs in the cities, while actually becoming prostitutes. After gaining some experience, these girls might join the army of migrant prostitutes, going to Hong Kong, Taiwan, New York, Tokyo or London with a work visa. After managing to build up savings, they might return home to get married or start a family business.

Migrant hookers usually arrive in Hong Kong having applied for a visa to make a family visit, take part in a group tour, receive medical treatment, go on a pleasure or business trip or participate in some other legitimate activity.

In the other direction, Hong Kong-based pimps representing organised prostitution go north to recruit girls under the guise of tour guides offering holiday trips to Hong Kong. It is generally possible to obtain only short visas but they do not want the risk of harbouring the girls in Hong Kong without one. This organised 'abduction of women' is based on a loose agreement; the northern girls work as prostitutes in designated places within the valid visa period. They accept recruitment by the pimps because the visa application needs a sponsor and the girls are not familiar with the customs procedures. In addition, they need basic information about living and accommodation in Hong Kong.

Even though the girls may have paid 10,000-20,000 RMB, which would normally secure a three-month visa, there is no guarantee they will not be apprehended by the police the very next day and repatriated. Despite this risk, northern girls do not fear arrest by Hong Kong police because they do not confiscate their earnings from prostitution. On the mainland, however, arrest invariably means confiscation of their money.

Deportation is also not seen as a threat as they plan to go home anyway. In fact, it is mainland customs officers who have stopped a number of provocatively dressed women from entering Hong Kong. Once, an officer at Lo Wu customs point, on the northern border of Hong Kong, was confronted with a group of 20 female tourists. None could speak Cantonese, but they all held visas issued by Heyuan County in Guangdong Province, where Cantonese is the spoken dialect. This discrepancy caused the officer to block their entry into Hong Kong.

Northern girls are normally able to obtain seven-day visas. During this short period, they exert all their energy and guile to attract customers in the street, in nightclubs, karaoke lounges, one-woman brothels, and porno internet cafés. Each minute represents potential income. Work first; rest second. There can be no private life. Trips are timed to avoid menstruation. They work from morning till night; maybe they try to snatch a nap in a clock hotel, then try to hook an all-night customer to save accommodation rental during their seven-day stint.

Rural girls from Hunan, Sichuan and Guizhou provinces charge only 20RMB in China, very different to what they can earn in Hong Kong. Seeing dollar signs in their eyes, they are delighted to serve any customer, and play any sex games.

Hong Kong prostitution has always observed unwritten rules. Streetwalkers will not undercut their peers. Hookers working in neighbourhoods do not bait or disturb local citizens but wait outside a clock hotel. Northern girls, however, have no time for these conventions and will pick up anyone they can, anywhere, at any price. They work bus stops, hardware stores, locksmiths, petrol stations, lorry drivers' rest areas, dockworkers' compounds, and anywhere else there are likely to be men. Older customers with a special appetite for street hookers have told me that HK$300 will cover room rent and a pretty young northern girl willing to provide the full course of seven flavours.

Local hookers use the phrase "northern girls are killing Hong Kong" to describe their depression at being left waiting for work while it is taken from under their noses. As angry as local girls may be, there is little they can do other than curse the northerners to anyone who will listen. They may try to scare local customers: "You want to fuck a northern girl? Just 50 bucks, maybe even including the whole night. Maybe you want to die young? One night with a northern girl will be your last, because they don't use condoms." Or, "Each time they come over, they fuck till their cunts are rotten. You want to stick your dick in that mess?" And, "They begin fucking the minute they get off the train; from seven in the morning until four the next morning. They must have steel pussies."

Portland Street is Hong Kong's infamous, cheap red-light district, and remains the prime target for Hong Kong police raids. Hookers would once complain liberally whenever the police mounted an anti-vice raid. Now, however, because of the competition from northern girls, local hookers want the police to come and sweep the northern girls off the street.

Some high-class northern girls work the nightclubs, but from the outside. They loiter around the nightclub entrances and solicit customers about to enter. Northern girls as 'nightclub take-out' are extremely popular because they only charge a few hundred dollars. This saves the customers from paying for hostesses' work hours, drinks, and buyout fees. Hong Kong nightclubs have suffered significantly from this poaching of their customers in the weak economy; some well known, longstanding nightclubs have even declared bankruptcy. Some madams experiencing a dramatic drop in business inside their nightclubs have actually become agents for 'northern girl take-out' by arranging customers for the girls by phone, and finding fresh northern girls to meet the demand.

I've witnessed the shocking difference in behaviour between northern girls and Hong Kong girls in the hostess lobbies of two nightclubs. Northern girls sit elegantly, looking decent and graceful, and seem well educated. Hong Kong hostesses, on the other hand, hang around killing time, gossiping and playing drinking games, or they sit with vacant expressions, like idiots taking a nap. While northern girls take pride in their appearance, and invest in their dress and coiffure, Hong Kong hostesses seem to have only a few evening dresses which are worn like uniforms.

Northern girls usually talk about sexual hygiene and health, while Hong Kong girls' conversation revolves around loans, gambling debts, lovers and husbands. Northern girls make an effort to stimulate a customer's interest and lust, and push for a sex deal. Hong Kong girls' attitudes can be less focused and more fickle. During the daytime, northern girls try to use their time profitably, and work the streets or hotel lobbies. They may pick up seven or eight customers during the day, helped by their bargain prices. Hong Kong girls seem more interested in sleeping and playing mahjong, and have little interest in doing much before 9:00pm. From a professional perspective, northern girls are obviously more businesslike and manage themselves more efficiently, while Hong Kong girls are more likely to concentrate on attending to lovers, having fun, and pampering themselves.

Visiting mainland businessmen, and rich mainland men who have permanent residences in Hong Kong, are generous patrons of the Hong Kong entertainment industry. They all prefer their fellow northern girls and appreciate their professional service. One madam said: "Each time I send out a local hooker, they'd have her replaced, disparaging her for her lack of professionalism, poor conversation, average looks but not-so-average price. So to cater for mainland customers around each national holiday, I have to try and stock up with a few extra local hookers willing to work for the price of northern girls."

Since Hong Kong financial secretary Antony Leung married Olympic medallist beauty Fu Mingxia, who was born in Wuhan, local customers have developed a sudden craving for Wuhan women. Many northern girls play on this and tell customers they are from Wuhan. A one-woman brothel simply put up a signboard reading "Hubei Fu Mingxia", which was later changed to the name of a movie star: "Hubei Zhang Ziyi", then to "Xinjiang Hottie", then simply "Mongolian Slut". This type of promotion indicates that northern girls not only sell their beauty cheaply, but also understand the attraction of exotica.

Although under fire from northern girls, local hookers are still preferred by some local customers. Those with a taste for northern girls might prefer to travel to the mainland to enjoy the wider choice on offer. They believe northern girls in Hong Kong, under pressure from their short visas, may take risks for a quick buck, which is associated with a higher chance of encountering an STD. Some customers are put off by the overly professional, almost cool, manner of northern girls, which lacks the pathos they have come to associate with prostitutes. Giving business to a girl with a pitiful story flatters the beneficence of the customer, and some find this is a significant part of the pleasure.

A girl from Sichuan told me that the earliest wave of modern Chinese prostitution began just at the end of the Cultural Revolution in 1976. Sichuan peasant women, who were desperately short of food, travelled to other provinces to sell their sexuality and fertility. Some went to Fujian, where they found business was easier than elsewhere. The cheapest way to inform their hometown sisters they had struck paydirt was to send a telegram containing the minimum number of words: "good money, men [meaning Fujian men] stupid, come quickly".

Another girl from the northeast, named Happy, told me a similar story but emphasised that the six-word telegram was sent from Guangdong to Liaoning. It is not important who sent the telegram, where from and where to. The point is that telegram gossip reflects a particular aspect of the development of prostitution in post-Mao China.

Happy had longed to experience life in a big city, but had to accept the boredom of growing up in a rural family in a county of Liaoning Province. Finishing junior high school, she finally found her chance to leave when she met Little Cai, a young man from the city of Shenyang. She immediately dumped her childhood sweetheart, packed little more than a toothbrush, and left.

Arriving in Shenyang, she found that Little Cai had spun her a story and was in fact a migrant with no permanent urban residence. She had no choice but to join the floating population. On their first night, poverty-stricken Little Cai could not find anywhere comfortable to stay, so the two squeezed into a single bed in a doss-house next to the train station. The next day, they began to search separately for some way to survive. The slightly more sophisticated Little Cai had no provincial accent and knew how to deal with urban residents, so he found a job as a waiter in a restaurant.

Happy would hang around on the street, watching everyone passing by, excited at the hustle and bustle. She quickly adapted to the local style of dress and speech and copied the methods of girls working the streets. She followed their example to solicit single men. Coyly, in Shenyang dialect, she tried: "Want to have sex?" Her first catch was a big success; not only did the man respond, but answered in pure Mandarin: "I've only got 100 yuan. Is it enough?"

After two months working at the train station and in big hotels, she made enough to rent a house in which to live with Little Cai. Out of gratitude, he took good care of her and looked after the house. He would work till late into the night while she walked the streets. They would both return home at around the same time for their midnight snack. He was amazed to see how much she was earning, and now realised that he had chanced upon a superstar when he met Happy. He became more and more in love with her and helped her work by ensuring her health and picking up extra condoms for her at the government birth control centre.

She spent money on clothes and make-up, and managed to double her price. After six months she had changed her dialect into Mandarin with a southern accent. Picking on northern guys, she would pretend to be a Hong Kong tourist who had the misfortune to lose her purse. The ruse was successful and gave her a lot of business.

Happy's skin was fair and delicate. Little Cai knew her complexion was a real asset and was worried that it could be aged by the weather if she continued working the streets, so he did his utmost to have her recommended into the best companion dance hall in the city, but she quickly found she was intimidated by the brash arrogance of the customers and superior attitude of the other girls. To give her more confidence, Little Cai taught her a few English sentences he had learned during his time in the restaurant. But again she returned home downhearted. In comparison, the other girls were much more worldly and cosmopolitan and her handful of English phrases could not help her save face.

Little Cai tried to comfort her: "They are more experienced, so what? They sell sex just the same as you. If we don't have the ability to compete as equals, let's just think about making money. You can tell them you are working to pay tuition fees for overseas study." The very next day, she learned the meaning of the English word 'happy', and took it as her name. With this special English name, Happy felt much better. Soon, her glamorous looks and easygoing charm were to impress the madam owner, who was willing to promote Happy to senior hostess.

Happy truly matched her name, enjoying a happy and successful career in prostitution. After a few years in the city she had been transformed from naive village girl to confident young woman. During her time with Little Cai she learned to smoke, to dance, and how to dress. She had become street smart and knew how to deal with strangers. She even learned about modern interior decoration. She became happier and happier and divided all her income into four: one quarter for her clothes; one to send home; one for Little Cai to look after daily expenditure; and one for her savings.

Happy and Little Cai held a lavish wedding ceremony in her home village and treated the whole village to a feast, distributing cash gifts to each guest. She installed air-conditioners and heaters at her middle school in the name of Little Cai, and won the gratitude of the whole village for her generosity. Her fellow villagers prayed for her good fortune and blessed her marriage.

The couple returned to the city and continued to earn more and save more. Happy was able to send more money to her middle school to buy new chairs and tables. She felt her good deed was truly recognised when her son looked exactly like Little Cai, which was a relief, bearing in mind her work. Happy had returned to her village for the birth, and after the baby's full month celebration the couple went back to the city, leaving the baby with Happy's mother. Little Cai continued his job in the restaurant and Happy went back to the dance hall.

After giving birth, Happy noticed her nipples had enlarged considerably and customers were pleased to fondle them, but her breasts were also tender and swollen. Happy found the extra attention her breasts received to be uncomfortable, so she took a pragmatic decision and allowed customers to suckle her milk for a price. As her breasts were emptied, her purse was filled. Soon after, she was fully recovered from the birth, and went to bed with the director of a colliery. She realised that she no longer had the tight pussy of a young girl, and thought of her client's coal mine.

She knew she could not continue as before and would have to find another source of income. The mayor of her village told her in a letter that there was a vacancy for her at the elementary school as deputy headmistress. A pimp had also offered her a business opportunity in Shenzhen, which Little Cai convinced her to accept, while he put himself forward for the school position. He could look after their son himself and she could have a chance to broaden her horizons in Shenzhen. Before departure, he bought her a sex health book, telling her to practice *chi kung* to strengthen and tone her vagina.

Three months as a hostess in Shenzhen made her almost fluent in Cantonese. Because Little Cai was not by her side, she worked day and night: at a little brothel during the evening, in a hotel lobby during the middle of the day, at a foot massage house in the afternoon for a few cheap customers, and part-time in a sauna in the early evening. Except for occasionally treating herself to good food and brand-name clothes, she sent the rest of her money home. She filled every minute she could with customers and felt her time was wasted if she was not working. Although some customers appreciated her slackened vagina, she spent almost all her spare time exercising to tighten its muscles. Her one abiding rule throughout was to use a condom at all times, regardless of price.

Happy made another generous donation to the school in her village, which helped Little Cai improve the school further, and later led to his promotion to the region's political consultative office. He raised their child and turned their large house into a little palace.

After a while in Shenzhen, Happy met up with a Hong Kong pimp who arranged a three-month return visa to Hong Kong for 20,000 RMB. She teamed up with some top-class northern girls for the trip and quickly found she had a liking for the extravagant gaudiness of Hong Kong nightlife in the clubs of Tsim Sha Tsui. Finding a position in a nightclub, she saw first-hand how prostitution worked in Hong Kong, and her confidence was boosted when she saw the local Hong Kong girls. She was not at all impressed by their slovenly approach to work, and instantly felt superior. In her view, they didn't deserve to work in magnificent clubs in such a high-priced market. The local girls neither sat decently nor stood gracefully. They behaved like monkeys. They were indifferent and they slouched and shuffled. She thought they had as much shape, taste and appeal as a bitter melon.

One madam who entertained tour groups of mainland businessmen gave the best description of the difference between northern girls and Hong Kong girls: "There's an ocean-wide gap in respect of education, dress style, body figure, and sex appeal. However, Hong Kong customers have weird spending habits. They don't care if they have bought good stock or not; instead, they believe they should go for local produce, always thinking that they could get cheaper northern girls in Shenzhen. The principle is not to pay a premium price for something imported when it can easily be bought cheaper in its home market. Following this attitude, they demand local girls in Hong Kong. Even if they are of poor quality, customers will pay the local price and feel at ease with their spending. This is a common logic and it is understood by northern girls."

She continued, "Local girls are always derogatory about northern girls and are quick to run them down at every opportunity. In front of customers, they heap insults on their northern rivals: northern girls fuck like mules; they crave money and don't give a shit about affection; they are outsiders, and they steal our jobs."

Happy had been through enough in her life not to be intimidated by the Hong Kong attitude to northern girls. Business in Hong Kong was not good overall, but Happy found that she, personally, found plenty of work. Besides the local businessmen who visited her nightclub, there were fellow businessmen from the mainland, and the Japanese. She could easily pick up a couple of deals each night. During the daytime, she might try her luck at the Convention and Exhibition Centre in Wan Chai, where investors in mainland businesses were eager to find entertainment for visiting mainland officials.

If Happy found work slow she would hook foreigners, generally considered by prostitutes to be a lower class of customer. Although she spoke only a little English, she found foreign customers were a safer bet, as the police normally do not bother foreigners. Attracting less attention from the police meant Happy was less likely to end up on a police blacklist. In addition, her immaculate dress sense, perfect make-up and casual but elegant manner gave her an air of respectability.

She found it easy to initiate conversations with foreigners, and flirt just enough to be invited for a drink. After a few sips, she'd say: "I like sex. I'm one in a thousand". This direct approach seemed to whet the appetite of western men, who were willing to accept her as a prostitute and pay a courtesan's price. Once, a handsome young foreigner was particularly aroused when she said "I like sex." Although he bargained well, she finally agreed to settle for HK$800. The minute they entered his apartment, she began to undress. After ten minutes' fucking, she was feeling sore, so she excused herself to the bathroom to apply some KY lubricant. After another ten minutes the young boy finished, and had reached his climax while urging her: "Faster! Harder!"

As she was leaving the building, Happy saw a bachelor in the next apartment. She put on her practised smile, caught his eye, and repeated the same line: "I like sex. I'm one in a thousand." He bargained even harder, and they cut a deal for HK$500. That night, she had met two smart-looking foreigners, next door to each other, and made deals with both of them.

Every year, she would come to Hong Kong for three months. Instead of renting accommodation she would just find an overnight customer. Her three-month assault on Hong Kong would make her a fortune. Their hometown house was becoming grander as she sent back more and more money. She also bought a house in Shenzhen so that Little Cai and their son could visit each year. After years of sex, fun and struggle, Happy had seen too many tragic endings to the lives of other girls, and considered it was due to an aimless lifestyle with no plan for the future. Drink hard when the wine is fine and gamble when there is money; easy come, easy go. These doomed hookers usually had a habit of attracting ne'er-do-well gigolos who would eventually ruin them. Happy was a hooker, but she set herself the goal of building up her hometown. She drew strength from her vision of life with a caring husband and a lovely son. She saw her destiny as being either headmistress of her school or the local cultural director.

Happy had not made many friends. Competition among girls for the same business made true friendship difficult, and those who didn't steal customers would try to borrow money. Little Cai told her to stay away from these fair-weather friends. She was close, however, to a Sichuan prostitute who neither gambled nor involved herself in tragic love affairs. The two would practise *chi kung* together to keep their vaginal muscles in shape.

Four years later, I ran into Happy's friend on the street. She told me that Happy had tried to return to her home village, but could not adjust to the slow pace of life. To keep herself busy she opened a brothel bar at Shekou in Shenzhen, in a joint venture arrangement with a number of other prostitutes. Most of the customers at Shekou are foreigners, so she tried to employ English-speaking hostesses whenever possible. When the bar was short of girls, she would engage the drinking customer in conversation, lean forward, gently touch his forearm and deliver her killer line: "I like sex. I'm one in a thousand."

# 9

## FERTILITY FOR SALE

The view in south China is that northern girls are looked down upon and northern wives are trodden on. Here is the story of Limfa, a peasant girl who would normally have few survival options. Without a pleasing appearance, she chose not to be a hooker, but followed a survival strategy more helpless than prostitution.

It was a typical morning at 6:30am on Mongkok Road. Construction workers were gathering to wait for the site supervisor, who would pick the labour he needed for the day. Uncle Gin could not sleep and had arrived at 5:00am. He needed money badly and wanted to be at the front of the queue. He squatted on the pavement and prayed for the supervisor to come early; no matter what, he had to work today.

Carrying a document folder and wearing a grey suit and a big smile, Kwai approached the hopeful men waiting for work. As Uncle Gin saw the smiling insurance salesman, he immediately turned away. Old Keung was standing next to him, and before he could do anything to save himself, Kwai had locked onto him, saying: "Hi there, Old Keung, you should buy insurance as early as you can. You are only in your fifties, with no injuries and no illness. The monthly payments would be very low."

Old Keung was tired of the repeated sales pitch and said to Kwai, "I have told you many times, wait till I find a wife."

The regular casual labourers nicknamed Kwai 'the insurance Kwai' – in Cantonese the word 'Kwai' sounds like 'loss' and insurance sounds like 'sure', indicating that buying insurance from Kwai did not sound like a good deal.

Insurance Kwai instantly responded to Old Keung: "You've been talking about getting married for years and years." But Old Keung was running out of patience: "You think I enjoy being single! I just can't raise enough for the marriage. What can I do?"

Seeing Uncle Gin trying to slip away, Kwai called out: "Hey Uncle Gin! Why are you so hard to find? The only place I can find you is here, early in the morning!"

"Don't push me so hard!" replied Uncle Gin. "I haven't cleared my prostitution debts yet, and my wife is having a new baby." Kwai was shocked. "Haven't you had enough babies, Uncle Gin?"

Old Keung was amazed as well. "Your first wife gave you four children, your new wife already had one, and you want more? That must cost you a few dollars!"

"She's a tigress, she won't have an abortion no matter what I say, so what can I do?" Uncle Gin sighed with resignation. Kwai showed no interest in Uncle Gin's family troubles; he just wanted him to pay the money he owed. "Uncle Gin, I paid your last month's life insurance premium, plus this month's. That's HK$1,120 you owe me."

"I don't want the insurance any more, I'm giving it up," said Uncle Gin.

"Giving it up? How about your little boys, your little girls, and your young wife, what will they do? Besides, you've already paid the insurance policy for a whole year; if you give up now, you won't get anything back."

This made Uncle Gin uneasy. "If I can get some work today, then I'll pay you back by instalments," he conceded.

The construction supervisor drove his lorry along Mongkok Road and pulled over in front of the hopeful crowd. He picked out a few strongly built men, leaving Uncle Gin to plead: "I've waited here every day and worked for you for years. For old times' sake, please take me, I'm desperate!" The captain nodded and Uncle Gin climbed into the back of the lorry.

The job that day was to move bricks to the higher floors of a partially finished building. Uncle Gin loaded bricks into the makeshift lift at ground level and passed them up to the waiting bricklayers, who were listening to a radio announcer repeating an irritating news item:

> *"The Court of Final Appeal has reached its verdict on the residency of Hong Kong citizens' children born outside Hong Kong. Yesterday, those violating their temporary visas stormed government offices and attacked the police in a show of anger. Both those who have stayed longer than permitted, and illegal immigrants, are praying for an amnesty from the SAR Government. Most of the overstayers say they are not willing to leave Hong Kong."*

The constant repetition of the news item annoyed Uncle Gin, who yelled out: "Hey, switch the channel, will you? I'm sick of hearing this news over and over again!"

While looking upwards and shouting, he lost his footing. The weight of the bricks he was carrying made it impossible for him to keep his balance. He toppled over and fell silent. An ambulance rushed to the scene, only to find Uncle Gin already dead amid a scattered load of bricks.

Limfa arrived in Hong Kong by ferry, holding her son in her arms and carrying an unborn baby in her belly. The crowded customs hall smelled of peasantry. She noticed a well-dressed, apparently educated lady and coyly followed her into one of the long queues. When Limfa was standing in front of the immigration officer at the head of the queue, she was suddenly inspired to tell him: "I came for my husband's funeral. My cousin saw me suffering so much, and she took great care of me." She looked past the officer towards the well-dressed lady. The officer turned and glanced at the supposed cousin and let Limfa enter.

Burdened with packages, suitcases and her son, Limfa came out of the customs building to look for her husband's family, who were nowhere to be seen. Then it began to rain heavily, which started the little boy crying.

Limfa watched the well-dressed lady get into a taxi while she cursed her in-laws: "The whole family are bastards! They don't care, they just want to abandon us, a poor widow and her child!"

It was now dark and Limfa stumbled towards her in-laws' house, struggling with the infant and her luggage. She could tolerate having no one meet her at the ferry terminal, she could even tolerate the rain; but nagging at her most was wondering how much funeral gift money the in-laws had received. She had calculated the number of his friends and relatives who might have attended her husband's funeral, and was expecting to receive a minimum of HK$9,000.

When she finally arrived, her first words to the several generations of female relatives seated at the dinner table did nothing to endear her. "Is the mourning ended now? Couldn't you wait a few more days to hold the funeral? What are you doing now, finishing off all the food gifts? How much money did you collect? It's my husband that died; all that money belongs to his widow and son!"

Without looking up, her sister-in-law spat out a fish bone and sneered to another family member: "Last time Limfa came to Hong Kong, she walked in and asked why there was only 10,000 dollars for the bride price. We told her, her husband's first wife didn't get a single cent from her wedding, so why should she be any different? Now she's after money again, this time from the funeral."

The little boy began to cry again, and the hard looks from the in-laws added to the palpable tension. Limfa began to weep: "You are all so mean. You just couldn't wait for a few more days."

The eldest daughter of Uncle Gin's first wife took a sip from her drink and said: "The funeral parlour charged daily and we had to pay all the funeral expenses. It was up to us to decide when to bury him."

"What about the cash gifts? How much is there?" asked Limfa.

Her husband's third sister was sick of arguing over money. She tossed a handful of notes at Limfa's face. "Friends and relatives donated this money for the children of your husband's first wife. You take this money and you never, never come here again!"

Limfa counted the money in tears, paused, and then screamed in anger: "Only five thousand dollars! You can't bully me and my children like that!"

Her husband's sister was outraged. "You deserve what you get! Is one child not enough for you? You're having more? You're shameless!"

Limfa's mother-in-law was in her eighties and looked frail, but her quiet demeanour suddenly changed and she screeched: "You want more babies! You fucking whore! Even if you bear more of my grandsons, I won't take you into our household!"

Limfa retorted: "Your son was old, ugly, and had stinking breath. I served him obediently for his last two years. Now you treat me like shit!"

The first wife's daughter was infuriated, shouting: "If you despised our dad so much, why did you pressure him into marriage?"

This enraged Limfa. "I forced your dad into marriage? Ha! It was your dad that tricked me into this marriage! He promised to give me this, give me that; in the end, he gave nothing but his shit, and you lot!"


Inside a tumbledown building in Sham Shui Po, Insurance Kwai was breathless from climbing seven floors. He had run into an old hooker at a one-woman brothel on the third floor; she fondled his crotch, trying for a deal. Kwai said he wasn't interested, and that he was an insurance agent there on business. The hooker's expression went cold. "If you were in the heroin business, maybe I'd be interested," she said and let him pass.

Kwai finally made it to the landing on the eighth floor, where he found a peasant woman washing nappies in an illegally pitched lean-to. He gathered his breath. "Excuse me. Are you Wong Limfa, Mr Ho Gin's widow?"

"You know my husband?" Limfa replied, excited. Kwai nodded. Limfa gave him an unexpurgated version of her time since arriving in Hong Kong, and her opinion of her in-laws. For the past few days, she hadn't been able to eat or sleep, thinking of the mean-spirited family. Kwai took a break while half-listening to her outpourings. She finally said, "My husband was a bit of a loner, but he's been here for all these years; he must have some friends, and he has his relatives. They told me there was only five thousand dollars gift money! Do you believe that? How will his widow and children live on that? Can you help me get the rest of the money?"

Kwai took a breath: "I'm not a debt collector. You have a one-million-dollar labour insurance policy; you won't starve to death."

"The labour insurance payout is one million? My husband dropped dead, and the compensation is so small! Somebody must have cut a piece out of it!" Limfa exclaimed.

"Your husband was just a temporary worker, and you think one million dollars compensation is small!" Kwai was shocked to find that the peasant woman was greedier than the local Hong Kong women he was more accustomed to.

"At least I'll have 500,000 dollars," she said.

"Why only half?" asked Kwai. "You've become a widow, and you still have to support your parents' household?"

Limfa cursed, then said, "Before marrying me, the bastard said he would invest in my family's business, but after we opened the shop with loans, he told us he had no money, and my family was put deep in debt."

Kwai's instincts told him that this peasant woman was going to be a pain in the neck if he let himself become too involved. He produced some documents from his folder and adopted a businesslike tone. "Ms Wong Limfa, Mr Ho Gin bought life insurance and you are the beneficiary."

Limfa was overjoyed: "Really? How much?" She was now so thrilled she verged on manic. She spoke uncontrollably and sprayed saliva onto Kwai's face. Kwai wiped himself with a tissue. Limfa was embarrassed and suddenly realised that she hadn't invited Kwai into her apartment. "Sir, what's your name please? Come on in."

The squalid room was strewn with nameless clutter. Uncle Gin's portrait hung on the wall and the incessant squalling of an unseen child filled the room. Three stools were piled with miscellaneous items, so Limfa pulled another tiny stool from under the bed and handed it to Kwai. The baby's screaming suddenly increased in volume, which merely irritated Limfa, who said: "That dead prick was hardly the perfect husband. He lived in this shitty chicken farm for ten years, and owed money to the hooker next door!"

Kwai tried some friendly conversation: "Why don't you find a better place?"

"Moving house will cost. There will be four of us. I have to save up." Kwai was surprised: "Four of you?" Limfa pointed at her belly: "I've been examined; it's twins." Kwai couldn't hold back his laughter. "Old Uncle Gin, no money and no skills, except making babies!"

"So how much will the life insurance pay me?" asked Limfa. Kwai began: "The amount is US$20,000, about HK$160,000. But – "

Limfa was disappointed and cut in: "Just 160,000! Why did the bastard buy so little insurance?" Kwai said, "Because I knew his family situation, I always tried to convince him to buy more cover, but he wouldn't listen. As it happens he didn't even pay the last two instalments, and you almost ended up with nothing." Limfa was terrified. "So how much is the insurance now?"

"Don't worry. You are lucky I paid those instalments for him, so you have the full amount. All you need to do is pay back what I've paid on his behalf." Limfa grew suspicious: "Now my husband is dead you can say whatever you want. I only receive 160,000 dollars, and you are going to take a bite from my payout."

Kwai was angry and stood up. "Cut the crap! I'm trying to help you!" Limfa fired back: "Don't treat me like a jackass just because I am a country woman, you bully! What made you so kind to pay for him in advance?"

"You think I like any of this?" said Kwai. "Insurance agents really hate it when people stop payments after a couple of months. We've done all the work, made the sale, and then we get no commission. Your husband almost stopped me from winning this year's sales championship. Each year, I have to sit at the round table at the annual sales meeting to hear about other people making a million dollars of sales. This year it was finally my turn!"

Back in his office, Kwai searched for the phone numbers of various social welfare agencies. A few phone calls led him to a social worker named Leung Chi-ko who specialised in immigrant services. Kwai told Chi-ko about a poor immigrant woman living in Sham Shui Po whose husband had tripped and fallen on a construction site, and died on the spot. The poor widow and babies had nobody to rely on and had to live in a run-down building housing one-woman brothels. It was so sad! He asked Chi-ko if social services could help her apply for residency, housing and government aid. During the conversation it took Kwai only a few minutes to get all the information he needed to size up Chi-ko as a potential client; he intended to visit him very soon.

For the rest of the day, Kwai planned to settle Wong Limfa's life insurance policy. Calculator in hand, Kwai mouthed to himself: "Government welfare, 7,000 dollars per month; dead husband's compensation, one million; half in the bank, that will get her 2,000 dollars monthly interest. The four of them will be living in public housing, and peasant women always try to save, so her maximum monthly expenses will be 6,000; then she could spend 2,000 on an insurance premium each month; she's young, so she could have a 15-year policy. She could be insured for two million Hong Kong dollars."

Chi-ko was paying Limfa a family visit. He was sitting on the same tiny stool used by Kwai. Limfa crawled under the bed and pulled out another matching stool. The leg of the stool dragged out a mousetrap, complete with a struggling mouse. Limfa opened the mousetrap and dangled the mouse by its tail in front of her infant. Watching the dying creature, Chi-ko felt sick and couldn't go on with the conversation. When Limfa began to talk, she said: "It's not that I want to have the babies. Doctors say the wounds from my last Caesarean aren't healed, so it's a high risk for me to have an abortion."

Although he was young, Chi-ko knew enough of gynaecology as a social worker to try to persuade Limfa otherwise. "If the wounds are not healed, you really shouldn't give birth at all."

The writhing mouse brushed against the child, who was now scared, and started to cry. Limfa killed the mouse with a blow from her slipper and dumped it into the waste bin. The baby's crying became louder and Limfa became annoyed. "If you keep crying, I'll make you eat the mouse!"

Chi-ko had to say something: "You have such a bad temper. If you have more babies, aren't you worried you may not be able to cope? A newborn is a little person, who needs to eat, be cleaned, looked after, and nurtured. Do you have the patience?"

The hooker next door was entertaining a customer. The rhythmic creaking of the bed springs bothered Chi-ko. "This environment isn't good for the kids. You want them to grow up like this?"

Limfa cut him short: "Of course not! That's why I have to get a residence visa. I can only apply for public housing when I have a visa, right?"

The occupants of the creaking bed were becoming increasingly vocal. Chi-ko struggled to contain his embarrassment. "One widow with three kids; why do you want to live in Hong Kong anyway?"

Limfa retorted: "You think I like it here? My whole village believes I married a rich Hong Kong guy. How can I go home with two empty hands and two new babies?"

"A mother should think about her kids' future. How can saving face with your village match your children's happiness?" Chi-ko asked.

Limfa felt she couldn't reason with this young man. "You are so naive! My face doesn't matter a bit; but if I don't have face, my kids will be bullied! Whatever bad luck I have, it's better to take it in Hong Kong."

"So you think more babies will win more sympathy from the immigration office?" he asked. Limfa nodded. "I know dealing with the immigration office won't be easy. Last time I had a baby, the immigration office showed no sympathy at all; they couldn't wait to send me home! This time, I will show them two new babies!"

The hooker's bed was creaking to a faster rhythm, and the baby continued crying. Limfa shouted at the baby: "You useless shit! You hear that bed day and night, what are you crying about?"

"Listen to yourself now," said Chi-ko. "How will you deal with two more babies? If you want to have the abortion…"

"Shut up!" Limfa screamed, her saliva spattering Chi-ko's face. He cleaned his face and saw a glimmer of maternity on those tough, angry features. Limfa cursed him: "What's wrong with you that you don't want others to have babies? Watch out you don't have a baby without an asshole!"

"I am just saying that you have no family here, you are a stranger in Hong Kong, it might be more convenient for you to live in your hometown."

Limfa shouted at him again: "Are you dumb, or just pretending? The mainland is reinforcing the birth control policy, and you are telling me to go back?"

Soon after Chi-ko left, Kwai arrived. Sitting on the same stool as before, Kwai took out an insurance plan tailored for Limfa, who was trying to feed her son porridge. She grew impatient: "Eat this, you sick son of a bitch! Or I'll throw you out onto the street!"

Kwai had never seen a mother behave this way before. However, she was his client, and a client is of course always right. He listened to her account of Chi-ko's visit and tried to take her side: "If he tells you to have an abortion again, you just talk about human rights! Anybody has the right to be born. Abortion is the murder of a little life!"

Feeling some emotional support, Limfa became more reasonable. "The social worker worried that I may not be able to handle it all by myself, but if I don't keep the babies, can he handle the immigration office for me? In Hong Kong everybody has to depend on themselves."

Kwai didn't know what to say, so he continued on the subject of insurance. "I've done some calculations for you. If you get government aid and public housing, you could make monthly savings." Limfa was delighted: "Excellent!"

Kwai went on: "Raising all these kids on your own, you've got to make some savings. Our company's life savings plan is the best choice for you; it would be worth two million Hong Kong dollars." Limfa was immediately dispirited. "I thought you were a good guy, and now you're trying to talk me into buying insurance!"

"It's for your own good," Kwai explained. "Only small payments each time, and in the future, you won't have to worry about your kids' education."

Out of idle curiosity she asked, "Over how many years do I pay?"

"I have tailored this 15-year scheme for you," Kwai said. Limfa was shocked: "I've suffered so much to give them life, and I have to pay for their education over 15 years as well?"

Now it was Kwai's turn to be surprised. "Haven't you thought about education? You are having babies! You think you are laying eggs, and you can walk away from them?"

Limfa dismissed the idea: "In my village we say born by nature, raised by nature. My parents gave me a life but never gave me an education."

Kwai was amazed. "So that's your 'nature' plan!" He was disappointed and shook his head at the carefully calculated insurance policy, which was now just scrap paper. In the name column, he wrote down "egg-laying woman", and for the insured sum, he wrote "0".

A few months later, Limfa, now heavily pregnant with her twins, was shopping on a Sham Shui Po street with her baby son. She was attracted by a news item on a display television. It was Ah Leung shouting "Return our rights of Hong Kong residency" amid a crowd of people storming the immigration tower. Limfa watched Ah Leung in silence, profound bitterness welling up deep inside her.

It was on the anniversary of her wedding to Ah Leung that she first met Uncle Gin. She had come to hate Ah Leung so much that each minute was a new torture. She bought a bottle of mouse poison and planned to take it all, and then sleep soundly and permanently in the bed where she had slept with Ah Leung.

After only a few sips of the poison, Limfa was interrupted by her sixth aunt, who said if she did nothing else, Limfa must meet a Hong Kong guy she knew, as he was looking for a wife. Limfa recalled she was still feeling drugged later in the day and could not clearly see Uncle Gin when she was introduced to him over dinner. Now she was his widow, she still could not remember his appearance. In her semi-conscious state, she remembered Uncle Gin saying: "The other village brought women in trucks to meet me, which really stunned me."

Limfa had no idea how her aunt convinced Uncle Gin to pick her. After vomiting the mouse poison into the toilet, she was told by her excited aunt: "Uncle Gin promised to take care of you and give your father a good bridal price. Now it's all up to you."

It had seemed a much easier decision to marry Ah Leung, who had no hesitation because her father was from Hong Kong. Now she could marry a naturalised, true Hong Kong citizen. She had been torn between finishing the mouse poison and marrying the old man for a ticket to Hong Kong. Her aunt reminded her that the old man from Hong Kong had been brought women by the truckload to choose from; if she didn't make up her mind, and quickly, the chance would slip away.

With a belly full of twins, her son on her back, and a name card in hand, Limfa was asking directions to the immigration centre. Help was given grudgingly, and she had to ask again and again. After a series of bus and train rides, she finally arrived at the new immigration service centre, only to find a cold reception from Chi-ko, who she had kept waiting. Limfa pleaded: "I'm almost ready, the twins could come at any minute. When I'm in hospital, there will be nobody to look after my son." Chi-ko interrupted: "We are not a nursery."

"I have no Hong Kong residency, so the government kindergartens won't accept me, and the private ones are too expensive," Limfa lamented. Chi-ko cut her short again: "Hong Kong government rules require that child carers have a professional licence, and we social workers are not licensed."

Limfa sounded helpless: "I know you are mad at me. But babies are human too. Anybody has the right to be born." Fearing that his colleagues may think he had violated human rights, Chi-ko decided he should try to finish the meeting and send her away as soon as he could. "You ask your in-laws to look after your son for a few days."

"If they could help, I wouldn't have come to you!" Limfa wailed. "I don't know how I've survived for the last few months. That dead prick didn't even leave me a TV set or a telephone, and I've just struggled all the way across Hong Kong to find you for some kind of help!"

The situation certainly aroused Chi-ko's compassion, and out of sympathy he tried to advise her: "You can't even spare time to go to the hospital now. When you have two more babies, you won't even have time to go to the toilet!"

Her tears rolled down freely: "If you don't want to help, forget it. You don't have to lecture me!"

By now, Chi-ko's colleagues were staring across at the distraught woman and he feared they would think he had discriminated against a mainlander, so he immediately changed attitude and softened his tone. "I've submitted all your applications. As for the nursing, even if I gave you a hand now, it could only be temporary, so you really have to think of some way to cope for the future."

Limfa asked: "Did you make it clear that I have *three* babies?"

It was getting dark. Limfa found a phone booth at the roadside in Sham Shui Po. Her belly seemed bigger than ever to her, and she was carrying a child on her back. Getting into the booth was a tricky manoeuvre. She took out Kwai's business card and began to dial. The street noises made it difficult to hear and she had to yell at the top of her voice: "Hello, is that Mr Kwai? I'm Wong Limfa, Uncle Gin's widow. A few months ago, you asked me to buy insurance. I have decided to agree to your offer, but you must promise to look after my baby for a few days."

Kwai was simultaneously irritated and intrigued: "Just to earn a little bit of commission, I have to look after your baby! Perhaps you should look somewhere else."

A rough-looking man was standing nearby and was staring at her. As she left the booth, he whispered to her: "Hey, how much do you charge?"

"I'm not a chicken!" she said. But the man wouldn't give up. "I'll give you plenty of cash. I love sucking milk." Limfa felt shocked and violated. She shrieked: "I'm not just another cheap northern girl. I'm a decent woman!"

She eventually managed to drag herself and a few plastic carrier bags of her meagre belongings to a gynaecology clinic. The attending nurse couldn't find any record of her and demanded to know where the pre-birth examination had been done. Limfa said: "I had a check right after I got pregnant. It's twins. Since then, I've been eating well, sleeping well; nothing has gone wrong."

The nurse was surprised. "You haven't had any pre-birth examination?" Limfa said, "I've really had no time. But I take herbal soup every day to soothe the foetus. It'll be OK."

The nurse warned Limfa: "Our hospital has no record of any pre-birth check; if anything goes wrong, we cannot be responsible. When are you due?"

"Any time now, maybe in a couple of days," Limfa answered. "I've brought my stuff with me." The nurse adopted a professional tone: "Do you have any labour pains?" Limfa shook her head. "Have your waters broken?" Again, Limfa shook her head. "Our delivery room won't take in anyone without signs of imminent labour. You'd better go home and come back when there are definite signs." The baby began to cry, which added to Limfa's distress. "I've had to come a long way to get here," she pleaded.

"Next time," said the nurse, "don't bring the baby to hospital, there is nobody to look after it for you. And remember to bring your Hong Kong ID card." Limfa was drained of her remaining strength and became desperate. She cried out: "I'm not having an illegitimate child. Why do I deserve this?"

She went to the phone in the hospital waiting room and wiped her tears while taking out Kwai's card. She called him again. Baby in one arm, phone in the other, she begged: "I'll spend all I have to buy your insurance, OK? But please, tomorrow, you've got to look after my baby, please!"

Limfa put down the receiver and idly watched the news on the waiting room television. There was an agitated mob of young people, born in mainland China of Hong Kong resident parents. The protesters were angry and some were trying to breach the gate of the SAR government buildings, screaming: "We want Tung Chee Hwa! Don't take away our residency!" Those at the rear were pushing forward; dustbins and bottles were being thrown at the police. The iron railing around the government headquarters finally gave way to the pressure of the surging crowd. Someone had started a bonfire.

While Limfa was looking for Ah Leung's face in the crowd, her baby started crying. She shouted at the baby: "What are you crying for? I give you a life and then have to raise you, on top of all this other crap! You think I'm Superwoman?"

Just as the Tsuen Wan-bound bus was shutting its door, Kwai caught up with it. He was leading Limfa's son with one hand and held two plastic carrier bags in the other. Limfa followed him onto the bus, out of breath. After a few minutes of jolting from the bus ride, Limfa realised she was soaking: her waters had broken. She yelled, "It's coming out, it's killing me!" This sent Kwai into a panic. All he could do was say: "Hold on! We are not at the hospital yet."

Limfa screamed in pain: "I can't take it, get the doctor!"

Kwai could see her agony. Her son was crying more loudly than ever. Kwai shouted to the bus driver, "Don't stop, this woman is going into labour, it's twins, it's three lives!"

The driver and passengers replied with one voice: "She's giving birth, and she's taking the bus! Just to save the taxi fare?"

Limfa's screeching upset everybody on the bus. One passenger came up and said she was a midwife. She touched Limfa's belly and looked nervous. She said to Kwai, "Your baby may not wait till we get to the hospital." Kwai immediately denied that it was his wife, or his baby.

The acute pain convinced Limfa that the bus was going to be her deathbed. She made a huge effort and grabbed Kwai by the sleeve, pleading: "I beg you, if I die, look after my baby, please, promise me!" Kwai nodded, under the gaze of the onlookers.

The pain had rendered her semi-comatose, in which state she thought she saw Ah Leung. "What is happening to us?" she thought. "You and your wife demonstrate in the streets for your right of residence, and I have to go into labour on a bus for mine!"

Telling the male passengers to stay away, the female passengers did what they could. After the first baby appeared, Limfa cried out in pain: "There's still the other one yet!" The bus finally made it to the hospital gate, where a medical team with a stretcher trolley were waiting.

It was early morning in Sham Shui Po. There was a huge pile of refuse waiting for collection on the street corner. Kwai and Chi-ko helped each other carry an old bedstead out from the dark old building, while Limfa, who had tied her twins to her back and her front, led her eldest son by one hand and carried a suitcase in the other. The local street hookers watched Limfa in envy and started their gossip: "Uncle Gin's wife made such a fuss about giving birth, she got everyone's sympathy." "I heard the government has given her a big apartment." Another said, "Sounds like I need to have a few babies to get the same benefits." Her friend replied, "What benefits? Her husband just upped and left after sowing his seed."

Chi-ko and Kwai laid the bed frame in the removal lorry and went back in for the remaining pieces of old furniture. Just then, the street hookers spotted several girls on the other side of the street. "Shit! Another group of northern girls! Trying to snatch our business this early in the morning!"

Limfa placed her suitcase in the lorry and seated her son next to the driver. She turned to see her fellow country girl Ah Liu standing in front of her. Limfa was delighted. "Hey, Ah Liu, I've made it! I've got my residency, government aid, and I'm moving to a new house!"

Ah Liu was not so delighted. "Since you sent home half a million dollars, everybody is expecting me to send home more money. My parents' face is all down to me."

Limfa said, "For me, living in Hong Kong is like a jail term." She suddenly saw the northern girls behind Ah Liu and realised. She asked Ah Liu: "Are you with them?"

Seeing the contempt in Limfa's expression, Ah Liu didn't reply, and took out some sweets to give to Limfa's little boy. Instinctively, Limfa blocked Ah Liu's hand from touching her son.

Ah Liu was hurt and walked away, saying: "Maybe I'm selling sex. But at least I'm not selling my womb."

Limfa yelled after her: "Selling my womb? I have to raise them, and see them through school!"

Two years later, Limfa married another temporary construction worker. Kwai was the matchmaker, pairing her up with one of his clients.

Social worker Chi-ko is now a district politician. When I met him recently, we discussed the constantly full state of Hong Kong's maternity wards. It's reported that 90% of these expectant women are not Hong Kong residents. Holding only a tourist visa, peasant women from Guangdong and Fujian provinces are prepared to enter Hong Kong at the last minute, with no pre-birth check records. Compelled by basic humanitarian principles, Hong Kong hospitals have no choice but to accept them, leading to yet another automatic right of residence for a woman willing to use her womb.

# 10

# Pimps

In the make-up room of a big nightclub in Tsim Sha Tsui, the company rules were posted for all to see. One of the rules stated: "No talking among hostesses and male colleagues in front of customers."

Two types of male colleague worked in the nightclub: waiters serving drinks, and managers running the hostesses. Nightclub managers evolved from conventionally active pimps, who worked their girlfriends, and passive pimps, who simply lived off their girlfriends' earnings. The strict ban on talking while on duty is part of prostitutes' professionalism and encourages them to find pimp boyfriends elsewhere. This keeps the complications of their private affairs separate from the operation of their workplace.

Powerful traffickers of women – hooker captains, procurers, pimps, gigolos and gangsters – have lost their control over prostitutes. Prostitutes' agents and the management system in nightclubs have abolished the conventional ransom system and adopted a modern contract system. This allows an indebted girl to turn down customers she doesn't want to receive, and the brothel can transfer her debt to collection agencies for recovery.

A successful prostitute's agent must offer star treatment to the girls under his management. It is in his interests to dress his women well and look after their appearance and accommodation, to allow them to concentrate on clients. He will try to enrich their knowledge, improve their conversation, and generally find ways to highlight their charm and sex appeal. He is simply working as hard as he can to develop the earning potential of his assets. However hard he tries, he cannot change the fact that only a very few of these cash cow candidates will become superstar earners. A successful agent needs to be skilled in keeping his superstar should he find one. Some will use their own money to lure the girl with attractive loans and commissions; others invest with affection, flattering the girl constantly to retain her loyalty. Others may use tricks to sow discord between a hostess and her agent so he can arrive in time to attract her away to his own stable. It's old news among Hong Kong luxury nightclubs that a madam is likely to be tracked down and punished for stealing a girl, while a club manager might be sued for snatching away a star hostess.

Nightclub male managers, known by prostitutes as 'daddies', share the same responsibilities as female managers, known by prostitutes as 'mamas'. Both daddies and mamas promote hostesses to customers like a property agent would promote an apartment, and charge commissions for each transaction. Daddies and mamas manoeuvre within the triangle of company, hostess and customer. Their job is to manage this complicated relationship, defuse confrontations, accept frequent bullying, and deal with the fact that 'the customers are always right'. It is not an easy matter to represent the interests of three parties to the satisfaction of all concerned.

Despite the necessary self-control shown by their agents, hostesses become more spoiled each day. They insist on increasingly luxurious treatment, demanding more and more from daddies and mamas, who in turn whine about being born into the wrong era. They yearn for the past, when hostesses were more humble, and more willing to take guidance.

Madam Dely became outraged at the mention of her star hostess. "Showing off her appearance, she would only pick the salty, soggy customers [customers obviously interested in sex and little else]; and once she was bought out she would immediately push for a sex deal, then come back for more. I'm not a one-woman brothel owner. How can I find so many customers for her to fuck?"

Madam Melissa shared her complaint: "My golden pineapple [the most popular hostess] will call first to see if there's a soggy customer to buy her out, and will only come in to work if there is one. She thinks her pussy is laced with gold, and she expects sex-starved customers to wait in line for her. But those eager fuckers won't wait for one second. Then, this golden pineapple blames me if she sees her customers fucking someone else."

Madam Stella said, "I understand that girls want to make quick money, and I try hard to tolerate their violations of the company rules. However, I really can't figure out why they squander their hard-earned money on gigolos; and they push customers to buy them out when they are out of cash. They're often dumped by their boyfriends. They end up in the casino, chain-smoking, looking like fishwives. They are not humans; they are scumbags."

Manager daddy Wong told me: "I earn my living from hostesses and I'm not supposed to talk about them behind their backs. But I'll tell you a simple truth: the reason they end up being hookers is because they are just too lazy to do anything else, even too lazy to give customers a friendly greeting."

Madam Debora had no popular hostesses, and the ones that were bought out often moved on to other clubs. Because the hostesses had no customers, madam Debora had no income. The club management told her to think of something to bring in some business, so she decided to improve the make-up and hair of the hostesses, to make them more appealing. However, all that happened was that the girls came to work with untidy hair, to take advantage of the free makeover. Every day, Debora had to fix bad hair and plain faces, which even then might not sell. I spent a few nights in the club and would hear her repeatedly scold hostesses in the same way: "You stupid bitches! You stink, why don't you use deodorant! You are too lazy to be a chicken, so how can you expect to be treated as a person?"

I also spent a few days in the lobbies of two other nightclubs watching mamas coach their hostesses in good manners and social diplomacy, and how to develop confidence in providing physical services to customers.

Apple was uncomfortably tense when she first joined the profession, with stiff movements and stilted conversation. Her customers would complain to madam Monica: "I came to spend money, not to rape someone." Monica felt Apple was not cut out for the work and tried to persuade her to change profession. However, Apple was desperate for money, so she carried on working with gritted teeth. Within two years, she had learned to relax but had gained an offhand manner. Again, customers complained to Monica, but for a different reason: "I came for a girl, not to throw cash in a plastic bag."

To best cater for most customers' tastes, girls need to play 'the inexperienced wild slut'. This requires an ability for role-playing that would severely test any professional actress, who would be hard pushed to play nine roles a year. A top hostess, however, could play the same number each day, with acting so real in order to adapt to customers whims, it would convince anybody. After the acting comes the actual sex.

Monica said: "Once in bed, even the least-experienced jackass hostess can get by without my instructions." She then reflected, "I wish sex work demanded good training. That might make the girls respect their profession, and then they would naturally respect themselves."

Being a successful prostitute's agent means adopting modern management techniques, revising the traditional image and becoming a professional 'horseman' – fashionable Cantonese slang for pimp. Fatty Dragon is a celebrity among horsemen.

Fatty Dragon writes about prostitution for several tabloid newspapers. His copy is typified by vulgar content in blunt street language, making it extremely popular among the Hong Kong male working class. For the last ten years, he has written for Hong Kong's bestselling *Apple Daily* and *Oriental Daily*. His column, 'Fatty Dragon Erotica', is often positioned next to the horse racing coverage, so that readers can review the sex market and racing form in one glance. Maybe Fatty Dragon himself is a gambler, which is why he uses horse racing imagery in writing about prostitutes. When he talks about a hooker, he will often use phrases like "a good horse", "a smart horse" or "a silly horse". He will describe a cheap establishment as a "horse stable" or "horse barn". He might describe nightclubs as "horseable intercourse", meaning one can be sociable with the horses and then have sex with them. He takes his time to evaluate the horses and barns in order to recommend good prospects and introduce new treats; he is, therefore, an expert "jockey".

Fatty often describes girls as "items", indicating that in his view, women are commodities. Similarly, advertisements for sex services in Hong Kong might state: "Wide variety of girls in stock, multiple choice, at sale prices."

To recommend the most intoxicating, cost-effective, innovative, smart-looking women and sex premises, Fatty Dragon needs to test the services on offer, rather like a chef must taste various cuisines to develop his own menu. Girls dare not offend Fatty Dragon and are prepared to line up to flatter and please him. Many offer themselves free of charge, hoping to be promoted in his column.

In his internet column, Fatty Dragon has said that with expensive hookers, he would sometimes actually have to pay; in contrast to the frequent free services given in return for recommending middle- and low-class brothels and individual girls. His remarks on expensive prostitutes never seem as enthusiastic as when he talks about cheap chickens.

There are so many prostitutes, nightclubs and bars in Hong Kong, and Fatty is only one man. He has claimed that others have used his name to obtain complimentary sex.

Using his huge popularity, Fatty Dragon joined forces with a multimedia conglomerate to publish *Hong Kong Nightlife Weekly* and an associated website. The constant flow of articles and pictures seems to capture the current state of the Hong Kong prostitution business, while providing some insight into the social aspects of the sex industry. When Hong Kong was discussing the implementation of 24-hour customs procedures on the border with China, Fatty Dragon predicted on his website that the new policy would have a disastrous effect on Hong Kong nightlife, and that business would migrate to the Pearl River Delta.

This northbound move would have a direct impact on Hong Kong's sex industry, and indirectly influence Hong Kong's economy.

When Hong Kong's Financial Secretary was announcing his annual budget, Fatty Dragon used the HK Nightlife website to attack the SAR government for not following the "One Country, Two Systems" policy of "allowing horse racing and dancing to carry on as normal". This would hurt the livelihood of the middle class which would, in turn, deal a direct blow to the sex industry. Fatty Dragon called for the whole industry to protest against the budget. In regard to the official anti-vice policy, Fatty Dragon wrote emotively about newly-pitiful chickens and accused the government of persecuting disadvantaged groups. As a remedy he encouraged the sex industry to develop new services to save itself.

When the Hong Kong sex industry was suffering from the SARS epidemic, Fatty Dragon advocated that hookers should "put on masks instead of bras", and use disinfectant spray before fellating customers. He also recommended "Radix Isatidis dragon drill" to appease SARS panic. Radix Isatidis is a traditional Chinese medicine with anti-viral properties, and as we know, dragon drill is a particularly popular form of analingus.

The prolonged SARS emergency was a disaster for many prostitutes, brothels and pimps, as business dried up. To save the market, Fatty Dragon felt he had to sacrifice northern girls and the lowest class of girls. He wrote in several articles that SARS came from the mainland, and that northern girls were all from rural areas, with little knowledge of hygiene, and would take on any business opportunities. He claimed he had witnessed many northern girls' rotten vaginas and advised customers to go to expensive local hostesses and stay away from the high-risk northerners. The result was that for the first time, Hong Kong ran short of northern girls, who preferred to settle for cheap deals on the mainland than go to Hong Kong to be treated as lepers. Unable to supply northern girls, some horse barns had to suspend operations or even shut down for good.

The shortage of northern girls severely damaged the long-term interests of the Hong Kong sex industry. Seeing this, Fatty Dragon changed his position and began to promote the idea that most northern girls were from peasant families. This meant the girls were hardy, with naturally strong immunity, and had the least chance of harbouring SARS. To further boost the attraction of northern girls, Fatty Dragon tried to change the Hong Kong perception that they were simply money-making machines. He emphasised their emotional qualities and said that frequenting them was like experiencing real romance.

Years of involvement with prostitution have made Fatty Dragon a well-known figure. It is said that every day he receives many readers' letters enquiring about the sex market. Older men ask which types of prostitute would best suit them; students ask whether a virgin boy will be turned down; housewives enquire about how to find clean girls for their husbands; some readers from Guangdong province are curious about Hong Kong prostitutes' special services; and some ask how to find condom-free girls. Fatty Dragon tried to persuade the condom-free seekers not to hurt either themselves or others. Some readers ask for the cheapest anal sex or dragon drill service. Some say they like cunnilingus and ask Fatty Dragon to recommend a clean vagina. A few readers claimed to have tasted all kinds of chicken except for the super-obese, and where could they find one? This request defeated Fatty Dragon.

Readers from Taiwan and the mainland all say they adore him but cannot really understand his Cantonese writing, and ask for simple word-by-word explanations.

A woman reader named Amy asked in her letter: "You've been a horse jockey for years, constantly using prostitutes. How does your wife feel about it?" Fatty Dragon replied: "When I started out, I had to test prostitutes almost every day; of course my wife objected. But that was my job and I had no choice. She understood and didn't argue. Now, a new generation of horsemen has already taken over, so I don't have to do it myself any more."

Not many pimps, procurers or madams have the abilities of Fatty Dragon to win over women. He relies not on force or trickery, but on his pen.

The downtown area of the Hong Kong sex industry is based around Portland Street in Mong Kok, which is jammed with a huge variety of middle- and low-priced brothels radiating sleazy glamour. It is odd to note that in this obvious red-light zone, there are few foreign tourists. It seems to be operated by locals, for locals. Recently, though, signboards using simplified Chinese characters have appeared, seemingly to attract mainland tourists.

Portland Street is Fatty Dragon's base of operations. Enormous varieties of women, sex games, nightclubs, karaoke lounges, saunas, Japanese-style blow job brothels, clock hotels and and take-out sets are on offer. There is even a male host nightclub to entertain off-duty prostitutes. All have evolved within Fatty Dragon's principle of survival of the fittest, leading to a booming sex industry. Fatty Dragon has horses throughout the stables on Portland Street. He has developed the role of conventional, trashy pimp into that of a professional pundit.

In October 2003, a Hong Kong local news item reported that a customer had removed his condom and forcibly continued with sexual intercourse, for which four pimps subsequently beat him to death.

# 11

# SAME OLD BUSINESS: NEW PROFESSIONALS REQUIRED

There is little doubt that the massive shift in the format of prostitution in Hong Kong during the 1990s was caused by a unique series of events. The handover to Beijing presented competition in the form of an influx of northern girls willing to work more cheaply, and the associated ease of travelling to nightclubs just over the border in Guangdong. The availability of internet porn exposed customers to new ideas. The cycle of market boom and recession severely reduced the number of customers, which meant the sex industry had to respond with lower prices and greater choice. In addition, there was the importation of well-intentioned liberal notions of rights for prostitutes. These events forever changed sex work in Hong Kong, and the way in which individuals provide their services.

When judging an individual's suitability for a given job, actual job performance may not be the primary factor. In prostitution, figure, appearance and age provide the first impression and can be more critical. One glance is enough for a snap decision to be made. Instant judgment denies the individual the opportunity to show his or her actual worth and ability, and serves to undermine self-confidence. Prostitution would appear to be an obvious case of this sort. However, in the context of commercial sex, traditional Chinese prostitution allows less obvious talents and non-visual assets to be appreciated.

Ah Ling, a hooker at the end of her working life, said: "Visitors to a zoo want to know the animal's pedigree, where its original habitat was, what it eats, and so on. When they look at hookers, the inner character, family background or life experiences are not significant; just one glance at the body determines their value. This naked stare makes average-looking hookers unwilling to tell others they are prostitutes, while the pretty ones brag about their booming business." Ah Ling went on to say that it is quite possible for average-looking hookers to have a lot of business, and sometimes earn even more than the pretty ones full of self-conceit. Ah Ling is one such average-looking hooker with good business, and does not readily reveal the nature of her work.

Her worst fear is not social discrimination, but the question "How is it you can sell yourself looking as you do?" When she hears this question, Ah Ling loathes herself. However, when given the opportunity to answer and recount her misfortunes, she finds that customers like to hear her stories, which she will embellish, inventing racy details. This is not because she wants to deceive. She simply understands that she has discovered her talent to satisfy a particular need. The man's self-image as a powerful and understanding benefactor is flattered. His ego is pleasured as much as his other parts.

In 1993, the *Sydney Chinese Daily* stirred up enormous controversy by publishing an article entitled "10 Western Men, 2 Mediocre, 8 Excellent; 10 Chinese Men, 2 Commonplace, 8 Suck." The columnist, a Miss Shi, was originally from Shanghai and married an old Australian man soon after she arrived in Australia. After she obtained permanent residency, she ran off with her French boyfriend. She hated Chinese culture but couldn't find any job opportunities outside the Chinese community in Australia. The article was her way of venting her anger towards Chinese men and Chinese culture.

The article outraged the local Chinese community. The next day, the newspaper's tiny office was jammed with 200 Chinese men, pressing Miss Shi to issue an open apology. She replied: "Apology? How can you have such an intense reaction? And why should I apologise for stating the truth?" These words not only infuriated Chinese men, but also Chinese women, who joined a campaign to reverse the perceived loss of dignity of the Chinese race.

The newspaper took the opportunity to sponsor an open forum on 'Chinese Men's Impotence'. Three hundred Chinese immigrants packed the meeting room. Many had taken time off from work or university, as earning a salary or studying for a degree was considered secondary in importance to repairing the shame caused to the Chinese community.

Miss Shi, having just lost her job, was alone in defending her position to the angry audience of Chinese people. She wept sporadically all through the event. With Miss Shi unable to effectively fight her corner, the Chinese audience felt cheated of a real victory. Carefully prepared, eloquent condemnations rapidly turned into personal abuse.

"Have you slept with all of us? What qualifies you to say we are impotent?"

"Just take a look at yourself! Who could have an orgasm with you?"

"You take a good look in the mirror, only ghosts would take you. How could any human being want you?"

"You shameless slut! Worshipping foreigners like a dog!"

"If you don't make an open apology to all Chinese men, I'll fuck your whole family."

The forum ended in farce, which attracted yet more attention from the media. It was reported that one Australian employer quoted Miss Shi's assertion that "Eight out of ten Chinese men suck" when criticising his Chinese members of staff. His remarks led to the resignation of five Chinese employees. Shortly afterwards, liberal supporters defended Miss Shi, saying: "Most Chinese men don't care much about their female partners' feelings in bed, so their performance is so-so. Western men highly value sexual pleasure, so naturally they make more effort and beat Chinese men in bed."

The point of Miss Shi's story is that the Chinese are often very uncomfortable with overt sexuality, especially in women, which is one reason why sex is traditionally camouflaged with distracting rituals.

Hong Kong people often blame prostitutes' outcast status on repression by feudalistic Chinese culture. Western anti-prostitution traditions have also condemned prostitutes and sexual hedonism, often using the Bible to support their arguments. By comparison, however, traditional Chinese culture was much more merciful to prostitutes, although not to sexual expression. Many folk stories feature romances between young intellectuals and girls in brothels. In these earlier times, Chinese prostitutes received rigid training from an early age in music, game playing, calligraphy and painting, and learnt the poetry of literary scholars and sentimental stories of heroines and heroes.

Not only have prostitutes supplied Chinese literature with many romantic legends, but they have also achieved positions of status and influence. Even the first wives of wealthy households dared not look down upon these prostitutes, and they would suggest husbands marry these wild flowers and keep them as concubines inside the family home for the sake of hygiene. The reverse situation appears in modern western culture. While sexual freedom is advocated, it does not follow that western cultural traditions tolerate the sex industry. Neither does western culture accept polygamy, and western prostitutes rarely integrate into large households as concubines.

Eroticism, as it exists in Chinese culture, seems to emphasise presentation over actual physical sex. In the same way that simple gifts may be packaged with fine wrapping paper and ribbons, so prostitutes present sex, with much show, play-acting and promise of what is to come. The stress, then, is on the art of prostitution, rather than actual sexual pleasure; on style rather than content. Furthermore, the use of prostitution is not associated with a particular socio-economic group. Consequently, prostitutes require the ability to deal with customers from all backgrounds with the same charm and grace.

There is a time-honoured idea of the prostitute as a social butterfly. A girl of lowly origins could work hard to learn the various graces and skills needed to entertain any of a brothel's customers. She had effectively achieved a new status that allowed her to accommodate patrons from all social levels, despite her own origins. It was an escape route from a potentially tough life and was tolerated as a career choice because it was recognised that this utilitarian means of survival provided support not only for the girl, but also for her family in the form of gifts.

Chinese men like to go to brothels to flirt with these social butterflies in order to satisfy their romantic desires, not just to scratch their sexual itch. They view prostitution dominated by sex as 'disgusting'. Prostitutes who have sexual intercourse with customers without flirtation must resort to accepting 'disgusting' customers. These are often older prostitutes who have no regular customers and have to work on the street or use a 'one apartment, one woman' brothel.

Chinese customers are classified by prostitutes as either 'romantic' or 'disgusting' while Chinese prostitutes are labelled as selling either 'art' or 'body'. Sex after flirting is the general practice of Chinese women who try to nurture a positive atmosphere with customers at brothels, nightclubs, bars and dance halls. The actual sex is conducted only after long-term patronage. The flirtatious prelude forces prostitutes to make great efforts to study make-up, manners and various dance steps, and to constantly enrich their knowledge to improve their conversation. They use their talents to adapt to a customer's requirements by acting as a dignified prostitute with a sad history, or as a feisty survivor in a man's world.

These girls are often quite ambitious, and regularly attend foreign language classes and hobby courses. Using acquired knowledge helps them to play the roles required by their customers. Although their job function includes a sex service, their role-playing ability makes them feel good about themselves as skilled social butterflies. In their own minds it helps them save face and maintain their personal dignity.

Many Asian women have a particular liking for western men, who are considered romantic and respectful of their lovers, and even tender and caring as one-night-stand partners. Yet, very few of the Hong Kong local prostitutes I know like western customers, claiming that their attitude towards prostitutes is not as respectful as Chinese men, and that they are mean and picky. The Hong Kong prostitution industry has always placed customers on three levels: high, middle and low, according to their style of consumption. Local businessmen fall into the high class, with Japanese businessmen taking the second position. Southeast Asians are also in the middle class, while western customers are deemed low-class.

The low ranking of the western customer is culturally determined. Typically, the westerner perceives a prostitute as a source of sex. They may show more concern for their partner's pleasure, but they are essentially out for sex, and want to maximise their sexual experience in the brief time available. They often have little interest in the slow build-up favoured by the traditional Chinese approach which leaves little time for coupling. Putting the priority on sex is the main reason western clients are considered low-class, and are deemed 'disgusting'.

The lack of emphasis on physical sex appears to be a traditional cultural imperative. Diminishing the sex component allows the girl to see herself as not just a sexual object, and therefore more than a mere prostitute; meanwhile, the man feels less shame on the basis he is there to appreciate the girl's grace, charm, personality and artistic abilities. It's rather like the man who says he buys men's girlie magazines for the articles on motoring.

Western customers speaking of Chinese prostitutes will say they had the impression that the girls were either putting off actual sex, or wanted it over as quickly as possible. This leaves westerners with the idea that Chinese eroticism is all suggestion, hints, pointless small talk and show, with little interest in the duration, quality or level of ultimate physical satisfaction. Oddly, the other general reaction by western men is quite the opposite. They find the coquettish approach and the stress on girlish femininity quite beguiling, because there is nothing like it in their previous experiences in the West. It represents a new experience compared to encounters with western women, who are more likely to be consciously or subconsciously informed by feminist attitudes.

The typical Chinese man appears to savour the non-sexual part of the experience, and has relatively low expectations about the quality of the brief sex he will finally receive. With regard to the sex, it is only important that he had a particular girl, who performed particular acts on him.

The East/West difference may be likened to a meal. The Chinese man wants every course available, or at least every course he can afford. He may also sample the restaurant's speciality whether he genuinely likes it or not, because he just wants it to be known that he is in charge and he has the money to pay for it. He will take all the complimentary tea, pickles and peanuts on offer. Somewhere during the meal, there will be a dessert course. The western man wants to get to the dessert course quickly, and eat dessert until he is stuffed.

Since the return of Hong Kong to Chinese sovereignty, mainland customers have seized the high-class position. Local businessmen, Japanese and Southeast Asians occupy the middle class, with westerners remaining at the bottom. The red-light zone of Wan Chai is a household name in the West thanks to the novel and film *The World of Suzie Wong*. Paradoxically, Wan Chai became an early Shangri-La for western sex hunters despite Chinese hookers' preference for Chinese customers. Even ageing hookers would rather work in a 'one apartment, one woman' brothel in the New Territories than hook westerners downtown in Wan Chai.

In order to continue capitalising on the Suzie Wong story, nightclub owners are reluctant to give up serving westerners who seem to have a particular affection for Wan Chai. So they conspire with human traffickers to import women from Southeast Asia as cheap girls for western visitors.

The western concept of rights for prostitutes was incubated under severe discrimination. Rebellion grows out of repression. So it is no wonder the prostitute rights movement has made remarkable progress in Europe and America. To uphold prostitutes' dignity, activists advocate the use of the term 'sex worker' – a politically correct term which stresses that being a prostitute is not only a job choice, but a valid one.

Since the 1990s, Hong Kong has witnessed a social movement to establish prostitutes' rights. Borrowing from the western experience, Hong Kong's social activists have pushed as far as they dare to advocate that 'sex workers' should enjoy rights equal to those of any other workers. As a result, customers began to develop notions of 'sex service', 'sex work' and 'sex workers'. However, the majority of Hong Kong prostitutes are deeply sceptical of this politically correct term.

Madam Monica at Club Bboss said that many nightclub hostesses in the 1970s were blessed with happy endings because they believed they were social butterflies who deserved rich men with high social status. To pave the way to their bright future, they were always busy upgrading themselves, and they needed to use their intelligence to demonstrate beauty and grace. These social butterflies lived in Tsim Sha Tsui in expensive rented apartments, not far from the nightclubs. In the mornings, they would invite regular patrons to their homes to treat them to rich cuisine. In the evenings, they would take the customers home to wine and dine them to develop an emotional link, then they would take the customers back to the nightclub. The girls were not selling sex, but their social graces and feminine wisdom and understanding should the men want to discuss their personal problems. During the day, they read newspapers and books to increase their knowledge, in order to provide intellectual topics for conversation with customers at night.

Even ten years ago, Hong Kong nightclub hostesses could still consider themselves social butterflies, respecting themselves, and attending to their dress and manners. Ambitious, they were still able to win customers over with their intelligence, playing the pitiful, downtrodden unfortunate while quietly planning for a happy new life.

The arrival of the term 'sex worker' stripped away the studied presentation and dissolved the mystique. It is a democratic definition, applied without discrimination to both the cheapest streetwalker and the most elegant social butterfly, who found there was to be no use for her intellect, artistic abilities or her skills at playing the roles of the modest ingénue or the pitiful unfortunate. Without these things, how could she continue to respect herself?

To survive, all she could do was drop the traditional role and go along with the new, blatant demand for novel sexual practices. With this transformation into the new professional, her customers started to forget the versatility and talents of before.

Since the notion of the sex worker has intruded into the sex industry, customers' attitudes have changed and they do the simple sum: which sex service is worth buying, and from which sex worker? The traditional practice of prostitution has turned into a straightforward business, just like ordering from a menu in a restaurant. In the intensely competitive sex industry, few sex workers can refuse a customer's order. The sellers' arts of seduction are deteriorating from lack of practice.

Now that the humour, romance, grace and glamour of the traditional rituals have lost their value, the role of social butterflies has been simplified into providing basic physical acts. They have been downgraded to sex workers, truly matching their new description.

Some nightclub customers are nostalgic about the fading memory of the traditional social butterfly, but now they can only find impatient hostesses who push for sex deals, with no skills other than offering pussy for cash. Once the hostess has dropped her mask to reveal her true nature, how can she continue to play the game of the 'dignified waif'? Not able to buy the courtesan experience, customers searching for the older style of service are often disappointed, so they are reduced to buying additional varieties of sex to compensate.

"Oh! Chickens today only charge with open legs!" Madam Monica said. She cannot forget the radiant hostesses of the old days. She said to me: "You wanna meet a happy chicken like Norma Jean Almodovar? Over ten years ago, I could gather up a whole basket full, any time. But these lousy chickens today don't even bother to ask the customer how they should address him, by his family name out of respect or by his given name. They are real sex slaves."

The blame for the redundancy of social butterflies cannot be placed entirely on Hong Kong activists. Why didn't the butterflies stand up for themselves, instead of hiding shyly in the shade?

One low-priced sex worker did not appreciate the respectful title either, as it demanded she be transformed into a new person. She complained: "To be a new person is to change profession. Who wants to be a lifetime hooker? Even if society were rid of discrimination one day, who would like to admit she's a sex worker? Because if we change profession and fill out a job application with 'three years of sex work experience', what kind of job can we find? If new employers refuse to hire us, the anti-discrimination agency can't sue them, because there's no way that sex work experience can help in getting a job unrelated to sex."

Who are sex workers after all? It is not just prostitutes who make a living from sex. There are writers of pornography, makers of pornographic films, glamour photographers, painters and their nude models, sex toy makers, aphrodisiac producers, sex doctors and therapists. Linguistic logic includes all of these.

Sweet-talking migrant Ah Ping was providing hand jobs in Mong Kok. She knew perfectly well how much men care about their penises. She would hold a customer's penis in one hand, delighted, admiring it as if it were a diamond. She said: "Men know it is flattery, but they still pay for the bullshit, it's well understood."

For the tiny ones, she'd say, "This is the perfect little bird to enjoy, the perfect size in the mouth, just reaching the throat, a real thrill!" For those a little bigger, she'd cry out: "I've never seen such a big dick!" For the uncircumcised ones, she'd say, "A real crown!" For the circumcised ones, she'd say, "What a beautiful shape, like a jewel! What lovely skin!" She would tell her friends: "Men are so silly, paying others to look at their ugly little sparrows."

The speciality of drug addict street hooker Lau Keikei was her first-class bed scream, with which she could convince anyone she was experiencing a staggering orgasm, an almost religious experience. To her, screaming and moaning was a distinct subject worthy of study, a philosophy. There were different performances for clitoral and vaginal orgasms, with variations for either continuous or intermittent orgasms. Once, she was in the right mood and demonstrated four or five types of scream for me in the street. It was so real, so thrilling, passers-by were obviously embarrassed, but fascinated and hypnotised.

Each time Lau Keikei sealed a deal with a customer, she would have to pay room rent by the hour. To save on her costs, she would scream and moan like a diva, the more sluttish the better, so that customers would finish sooner. She worked at training her bed scream to achieve ultimate perfection.

Sometimes customers thought she had real feelings for them. One old guy said to her with heartfelt sincerity: "If you hadn't fucked my buddy, I'd marry you." She replied, "You can marry your old mother! Give me a cigarette." Lau Keikei didn't give a shit.

Hong Kong prostitutes know how to use obscenity. In ascending order of offence, they would curse mothers, then fathers, and finally the ancestry of 800 generations. The ripe language flows easily, any time, anywhere; in bed, at the mahjong table, to people they like, and to those they don't. They pride themselves on an enormous variety of ribald and disgusting expletives, and amazing creativity in the use of them. They inject their rich vocabulary of vulgarities into local language, making Hong Kong Cantonese more dynamic. In the unfavourable Hong Kong sex market, under competition from northern girls, Hong Kong hookers' fruity language has served them well. Local customers, unaccustomed to such intense loquacity, find the shock value so exciting that they finish the business in a few or even fewer strokes, leaving them with no energy or inclination to talk to northern girls in their polite Mandarin.

What makes happiness? It's not money. Those who hate their work are the least happy, while those who enjoy their work are the most happy. Following this popular view, activists for prostitutes' rights promote the idea that if it is possible to find a way to enjoy sex work, the workers will become happier. The argument continues that if brothels are filled with happy girls making money while having fun, then the dignity, rights, legal status and tax contributions of prostitutes would follow on naturally. Those who can make money while enjoying sex must have the best of jobs.

Therefore, encouraging prostitutes to find a way of working that allows them to tell the general public that they enjoy sex while serving customers is a major part of the prostitute rights movement.

I asked many prostitutes: "Have you ever had an orgasm during work?" They all answered "No". One hooker retorted: "A waitress may sometimes have a good meal in the restaurant kitchen, but can you say she picked the job for the good food?"

I was desperate to find a happy hooker like Norma Jean Almodovar, and exasperated my informants with the repeated question: "Is there anyone who chooses to be a prostitute simply because she likes sex?" They were all bewildered that I should ask such an idiotic question. "Is there a chicken not working for money? Being a hooker just because she likes to have sex? Is there a lousy chicken like that?"

I told them about Almodovar, the Los Angeles police officer who gave up her career and chose to be a hooker, and they all said that Norma Jean was a "super bag of shit". Of course, in Hong Kong as everywhere, there are women who love sex, and these women can hook up with as many men as they please. They needn't put a price on themselves to enjoy abundant orgasms from sex, so why should they go into business and receive customers?

Prostitution is basically physical labour. Even for the most lustful women, once they become sex workers they become sex labourers. Can anyone enjoy an orgasm during hard labour?

My informants repeatedly emphasised that the only reason for them to quit the business was to enjoy sex with their lovers. The prostitutes' accounts of their lack of enjoyment are quite different to reports by customers published in *Call Girl Directory*. The men believe that the level of a girl's secretions is an indication of her excitement. Prostitutes, however, reveal they have two powerful allies: condoms, which are pre-lubricated, and surreptitious, unnoticed applications of KY jelly. Several hookers have in fact laid down a challenge: "If you find a chicken whose sweet talk was matched by a hungry pussy, we will chop our heads off for you."

The changes brought about by the combined effects of competition from an inflow of northern girls, the economic crisis, greater ease in crossing the Hong Kong/China border and the promotion of prostitutes' rights as sex workers have permanently changed the landscape of the

Hong Kong sex industry. The loss of the traditional coquette with all her artifice is balanced by the appearance of a wider range of outlets and demand for a greater range of services. It is possible to suggest that the initiative is no longer with the provider and has passed to the consumer.

As the relative price of commercial sex has dropped, control has passed from the gangsters, pimps and brothel owners to the actual sex workers, who have found that while they may have more freedom to operate as they please, they also have to compete as never before.

As with all products and services, increasing choice has a forward momentum. Nostalgia, however, can be instrumental in creating niche markets to bring back things fondly remembered. It may be, therefore, that the traditional style of Chinese prostitution eventually returns, in limited supply and at a price, as a status symbol for the wealthier customer.

# 12

# LOVE, FACE, AND THE FUTURE

## Love

There are abundant instances of prostitutes giving their money away to their lovers. Why do they seem so willing to give their money, earned from men, to other men? How much emotion is involved in the money? How much love? In *Prostitutes' History*, the only book about prostitution approved by the Chinese government, there is a vivid description of sports activities enjoyed by traditional prostitutes, but little about their emotional lives. It would seem they don't deserve love. In fact, their love is often the most naive and intense in nature, typically ending in tragedy.

Prostitutes have a stronger desire for love than do average women. Sexually, the female body is more complex than the male, and arousal can be more intense and prolonged during an intimate physical encounter. Customers can simply walk away when the business is done, but if the prostitute has become genuinely aroused, she must cry inwardly while watching her paramour leave. To keep emotion out of business, prostitutes must make a clear distinction between lovers and customers. The body is a business tool, which has to be touched by many customers; lips are the forbidden area reserved for lovers. However, because of aggressive competition, Hong Kong hookers have already sold their kisses as sex treats.

Many prostitutes come from problem families, often lacking in affection. Like Lau Keikei, they are love-starved patients. Madams and managers all coach prostitutes with the same sex theory: those who can save enough and walk out of the business are free from emotional trouble; those who become involved will definitely suffer heartache, mental distress, and possibly depression.

Because of their desperate need for love and approval, prostitutes appear to show little discrimination in their choice of lovers. They often entrust their life, joy and money all to their beloved men. Once in love, they are unlikely to stop and consider whether their lover might be overwhelmed by such generosity. To lavish all on an individual may be an attempt to balance personal karma, to counteract the culturally perceived and actual negative aspects of sex work.

The common assumption is that procurers, pimps and gigolos are exploitative vampires. In fact, men preying on women have their own sorrows. Prostitutes have a joke that men must "Go home and pay tax to the jackal." Despite knowing the nature of the beast, they still choose to keep it at home. The taming of the jackal is a metaphor for dealing with a life of whoredom, and winning.

I interviewed the lovers of two prostitutes. They seemed more understanding than average men and had no self-evident prejudice against hookers. They understood the prostitute's psychology, and were willing to provide them love and support.

Ah Goo would drive his girlfriend to work on the Sham Shui Po streets in an old Mercedes-Benz. He would then go to buy her a lunch box. On one such trip I accompanied him and asked: "Do you really love her? Don't you mind her profession?"

Ah Goo sighed, "As soon as a man has a hooker for a lover, he's gonna be taken as a parasite living off prostitution. Actually, I have never taken a cent from her. I have even lent her money, telling her to change profession, but she's buying an apartment with a heavy mortgage, so I understand the situation. I don't look down on her for not changing her work because I'm in love with her, it's that simple."

Ah Goo respected her decision to delay changing profession, but this respect was misconstrued as evidence of living off hookers, so he intentionally drove his girlfriend to work in an ageing car to prove otherwise. After delivering the lunch box, Ah Goo became miserable again. "It's very hard to maintain emotional ties with prostitutes who are naturally suspicious of men; lacking confidence but craving emotions. If I ignore her for a second, she'll kneel down to beg me to treat her a little nicer, it's quite tense."

Another man was crazy for a Taiwanese prostitute. When she decided to get married to a different man, she gave him HK$100,000, telling him to find another woman for marriage.

Soon after taking on a job in a nightclub, Ah Ching met newly divorced Bing, who fell instantly and desperately in love with her, so much so that he gave her his share of his company's dividends. Ah Ching was thrilled. She vowed the feelings were mutual and that she was in love from the bottom of her soul.

Two weeks later, Bing had become resigned to her four phone calls a day. A month later, he was barely able to tolerate her needy, clinging behaviour. After six weeks, he said "Give me a break," which made Ah Ching panic. Her madam gave her some advice: keeping a man is like flying a kite. To keep him aloft, you must let the string roll out.

She just could not follow this advice and Bing grew colder, so she tried giving him increasingly expensive gifts. Bing's passion for her was gone, and he began to chase another girl. He needed money, so he demanded it from Ah Ching, who was desperate to keep him. She was prepared to trade cash for love and dared not walk away. She refused to see the truth and foolishly handed Bing all the money she made from prostitution each night. He was all she had; without him, she could not live, and as long as he wanted her money, he would be her man.

Having a woman so dedicated to him made Bing feel trapped, so he would abuse her whenever they met, just to get rid of her. Finally, he became hysterical and gave Ah Ching a severe beating. Afterwards he gripped her by the collar and yelled: "You are a real junkie! I can't even bat you away."

Ah Ching's love story is commonplace among prostitutes. Her love philosophy was to stay faithful to the end, until emotionally tortured to death by her lover. She wished she could have a little more luck and keep her lover with her. They might die together, or she might be killed by him. For prostitutes, love means death. Many prostitutes have had narrow escapes and have met other men just before they felt they were about to die, so they would be off on further emotional roller coaster rides. For someone in love with a prostitute, embarking on a relationship is like entering a battlefield from which no one escapes alive. To make a successful exit, they need to be cold-blooded enough to dump their prostitute lovers, who are themselves prepared to die on the battlefield in order to prevent their lovers' escape.

It is a fact that there are men living off women who they coaxed into prostitution; it is also evident that a prostitute's clinging style of love can be overwhelming. While some men feel suffocated and choose to get out, others stay and effectively become personal managers.

A prostitute's love is as doomed as that of a kept mistress, who is unhappy in luxury. Hong Kong sees many beautiful northern women in fashionable dress and jewellery, living in expensive residences, playing mahjong all day long. They are not housewives, but neither can they name their profession. I spent time with a number of 'second wives' and eventually learned they had moved from the *er nai* villages in Shenzhen.

*Er nai* are two Chinese characters which literally mean 'second wife'. The term was used as a form of respectful address in wealthy households to refer to the master's concubines. A new meaning developed in the 1990s, when another form of prostitution began to appear. Within such relationships, a man 'owns' a woman outside wedlock, and gives her money and other material rewards for her companionship and other services. It is different from other kinds of prostitution in that it is a relatively stable relationship and is longer-lasting. Some women actually have multiple identities because while they are *er nai* they are simultaneously performing other types of prostitution. This is because the men who 'own' them may not live with them, which gives them personal time and space.

The *er nai* villages in Shenzhen have been established for two decades, supported mainly by Hong Kong working-class men. Keeping a second wife across the border costs a Hong Kong man only HK$3,000 a month. For this amount, someone on a low income can afford to rent a flat in Shenzhen to accommodate his second wife, and visit her regularly.

Little Mi told me she was no ordinary woman and claimed she was doing the hardest job. Coming from the countryside in Hubei province in mainland China, she became a kept mistress in Hong Kong immediately after her divorce, planning to find a sugar daddy to fully support her while still young. A mistress makes herself available to only one man at a time, and he normally offers to maintain an apartment and a car for her during the relationship. Changing her 'husband' each year, Little Mi had been the mistress of three men. With her first she cried, fought, and even threatened suicide. After one year's effort on her part, the man paid only half the mortgage, then left for good. The second 'husband' paid for the other half then he, too, left. She schemed to cut a good deal with the third 'husband' and managed to gouge him for an additional apartment for her retirement. However, after she pulled off the deal, Little Mi fell in love with this third 'husband' and ended up a penniless 'second wife'.

This 'second wife' or mistress relationship is not based on love or anything similar to a marriage contract. From the emotional and legal perspective, the 'husband' is free to walk away at any time. The vital ingredient to maintain the arrangement is the sponsor's passion. Little Mi understood that male sexual passion is fickle, so she would play all the roles necessary to keep his interest: good housewife, coquettish slut, elegant lady, pitiful wretch and beautiful model. Even though she put on a new face every day, the money from her 'husband' dried up. When a 'husband' does not come visiting, killing time can be a chore. Second wives have a knack of finding women in like situations and they form their own circles. When they flock together, they speculate on who may soon be dumped and who is currently in favour. Once they find out that a 'husband' is cooling down, second wives immediately take note, so they might line up a replacement should they be abandoned. In order to survive, members of the second wife sisterhood can never be too watchful of each other's affairs.

Non-mistress friends may ask a mistress: "If you don't have much to do, why don't you read to improve yourself?" Little Mi's job was to dress up and look her best, and wait around the clock for her 'husband' to visit, while getting ready to fight for men with other pretty women; how could she have time for reading? Besides, it seemed to her that men paying for a second wife usually didn't like them to read very much.

Little Mi's 'husband' excused himself for ten days because his legal wife was keeping a keen eye on him. Little Mi could not sleep during those ten days. She was exhausted but just could not sleep, no matter how much she wanted to. Desperate, she locked her front door, closed all the windows, and turned on the gas.

She awoke in hospital to see her proxy husband's face, and thought: "The big wife should know how I've suffered." Then she saw her friend, Li. Her 'husband' said it was Li who had sent her to hospital. A short while ago, Li had asserted that she would not yield to the fate of being a mistress kept out of sight by a 'husband' who was beginning to lose interest in her. She borrowed HK$100,000 from Little Mi to buy a diamond Rolex watch in an attempt to impress her 'husband' and keep his interest. Li hadn't won back her man but was wearing a new pair of heart-shaped diamonds. Lying on her hospital bed, Little Mi thought, "I must keep an eye on Li".

Her 'husband' told Little Mi that his business was not doing well because of a cash flow problem. He asked her for a temporary loan, which would be paid back double. After several years as a second wife she had gained an apartment and HK$500,000 in savings. She gave him the money for his business. She could have driven a harder bargain but this time she was much more interested in his love than his money. The husband then avoided her, using the excuse that his legal wife was watching him. Frustrated, Little Mi called the legal wife and laid her cards on the table: "I don't want to break up your family, but you should know of my existence. I'm also his wife." The showdown did not improve her situation.

The legal wife brought over a bunch of rough women who gave Little Mi a severe beating. Without any sympathy, her 'husband' said: "You started it. You got what you deserved!" She suddenly realised that as a second wife she had no rights or protection. She wondered how the legal wife could have no idea that her husband's business was suffering, while she went on enjoying her mahjong. Why was it that the second wife had to draw on her savings to save the business? Because the man was in control of her love, and had lost his passion, he simply decided that before walking away he'd like to make some money out of her.

Many second wives are prepared to use their savings to help their 'husbands', with the agenda of retaining their love. Smart men know that after an initial extravagant gesture to gain her attention, the ongoing cost of a second wife is not that great. Providing she can avoid emotional involvement, a second wife can make a net gain, especially if she can line up another 'husband' to benefit from the initial investment in her when the previous one has lost interest and moved on.

For a second wife, emotional involvement can mean a reduction in income and a broken heart. It seems that few second wives have emotional immunity. If a second wife dedicates all her time and intimacy to the same man there is always the chance of an genuine attachment developing, unless her personality is flawed or she has her own lover unknown to the 'husband'.

When second wives talk about the value of money and gifts they receive from their 'husbands', figures of hundreds of thousands of dollars are often mentioned. However, I have seen very few second wives with any outward signs of wealth. In conversations between second wives, values are commonly exaggerated by a factor of ten. This habit of bragging is a major difference between second wives and prostitutes.

*Face*

Nothing is more tedious than 'dying to save face', but nothing is more important than face for male and female prostitutes. Some prostitutes develop a face-saving fetish out of an inferiority complex. In others it seems innate, in which case they need increasing amounts of money to maintain their face, and prostitution provides the necessary income.

One procurer took exception to my worn purse, saying "A man makes an impression and establishes face with his shoes, while for a woman it is her handbag. How can you allow yourself to be seen with such a shitty old purse?" Our value systems were obviously different. I had owned my handbag for ten years and was comfortable with it; it did what I wanted. My handbag may have been modest but it was not fake, it was just old, and looked it.

Ah Kuen claimed to be my "best friend". She invited me to dinner with her occultist. She praised me to the heavens in every possible way, and quietly suggested I pay the bill for dinner. When my token attempt at asking for the bill was thwarted by the occultist, Ah Kuen's face blushed as if it had been peeled.

On another occasion, Madam Dodo mentioned me while chatting with friends and called me to join them: "We would like to treat you to a midnight snack. You've got to come, or I'll lose face."

Warm-hearted Fanny, a madam, helped me arrange an interview fee with her girls, which stood at HK$4,000 to HK$5,000 after negotiation. I said, "I can't afford so much." She cursed me for my stinginess and claimed I had made her lose face. She had to justify to her associates why she was still spending time with me, making the excuse that we had other business. To justify the excuse she pressed me to poach hostesses for her from other madams, trying to motivate me with high commissions.

Sisley had a sister who had quit prostitution and opened a beauty parlour. She took me there to do my hair. As her sister was playing mahjong at the time, she was reluctant to receive us. While my hair was being done, Sisley bragged to her sister about how her boyfriend loved her, even though I had witnessed her boyfriend treating her badly. Then, Sisley boasted that several men were trying to buy her out of her club. In truth, the club was not happy about employing her because she was ageing, and she had been told she was becoming an embarrassment to both the club and herself. She had pleaded with the club to find her a job in a cheap brothel. After my hair was done, I was shocked when her sister charged each of us HK$1,000. This was a very high price for a local, family-owned beauty parlour. Sisley asked me to save her face and pay for both of us, with a smile. Because at that time she was still indebted to the club where she worked, she 'borrowed' a further HK$100 from me for a tip.

If prostitutes' love is a matter of life and death, then their friendship is equally extreme. Friendship to them is not so much an intimate affection between people, but more a matter of face, which is based on a dislike of arguing over petty details.

Prostitutes can be very forthright in friendship and will make up their minds very quickly. You will be instantly accepted or rejected. This may be because they have to maintain a sociable attitude in their work, so in their own time are less disposed to being polite for its own sake.

If you click, you have found yourself a most faithful friend. They will give their help willingly if you are in trouble or if you ask a favour. If you are bullied, they might even arrange for your aggressor to be beaten up. Repayment with money is frowned upon; money in return for a favour is too close to their work.

Their attitudes are summed up in statements like "I don't charge a friend" or "friends don't bargain". However, this leaves you to wonder what might ultimately be expected of you if they were ever in need. Indeed, if they ever state "I would do anything for a good friend" there is no telling what they might expect from the friend in return. If you are very busy and seem to have no time for them, you risk causing offence by placing business above their friendship.

A prostitute friend I had just made wanted to borrow money. I had no money and she could understand that. She wanted me to ask my other friends, who may have had more money, to help her. Another prostitute friend asked me to visit a hospital patient who I did not know. She said, "You've got to come. He cast a spell that backfired, so he is now suffering for somebody else's sin. He's a really nice man."

Even today, I cannot understand why Winnie decided we were the best of friends just after we met for the first time. One day, after her nightclub closed, Winnie wanted to spend the night with me. I said I only had a single bed, to which she said she could squeeze in. I replied I was not used to sharing a bed, and she called me a freak. Another time, very early in the morning, she called me over to have a drink with her. I said I had just gone to bed and had to work the next day. She became angry and said, "Aren't you my friend?" The next time we met she was cold, saying: "I'm a vulnerable woman."

Several madams told me that prostitutes hate making friends with well-mannered professionals. To them, a polite friendship is lukewarm, shallow and lacking in passion. Hostesses much prefer a rakish, devil-may-care man they can greet wildly, like a long-lost family member. Should they meet decent men, they will respect them by maintaining a cool demeanour.

It was no wonder, then, that the hostesses I met were invariably polite to me, and sometimes even took me to be a customer. When they found out what I wanted, they would say: "You can interview me, I will only charge HK$1,000 per hour." I told them that even a lawyer wouldn't charge me that much, and the disingenuous response would be: we hate to bargain, and we have very little idea about prices.

I was recommended to Fanny, who introduced me to Junjun. I had little chemistry with Fanny, but hit it off instantly with Junjun, who I was pleased to invite to dinner. She was delighted to accept.

Immediately before the date, Fanny called to ask if I had seen Junjun. I said yes, and Fanny blamed me for not giving her face, telling me that I had to go through her to meet Junjun from then on. I didn't understand, but understood later when Junjun stood me up.

Later, Fanny said she would find a gigolo for me to interview, saying that Raymond knew the gigolo business inside out. I called Raymond, who promised instantly to take me to a host club.

During the evening, Raymond told me that I should give face to Fanny, and that this was the rule. I felt the rule was rather unnecessary, but Fanny was truly angry, and when we spoke again she yelled at me: "You are my friend, but how can that be so when you go past me and directly contact my friends, making me lose face?"

*Future*

Prostitution tends to attract those with a taste for risk and making a quick buck; they have no patience for future planning and are prepared to gamble with their energy, money, and body.

Madam Melissa managed a successful hostess called Earn, who had the looks and grace of a supermodel; she had many admirers, including some very powerful businessmen. Earn had a habit of disappearing for days at a time. Once, Melissa visited Macau and ran into Earn in a casino. She looked dishevelled and her make-up was beginning to run. She took HK$300 from her handbag and pushed it across the blackjack table. The banker dealt the cards and Earn picked them up while squinting through the smoke of a cigarette butt in the corner of her mouth. She looked like a professional gambler as she picked up the cards and slowly and deliberately fanned them.

"Fuck! Fuck! Fuck!" she screamed as she saw her hand. The supermodel was now a maniacal loser. In her rage, she sprayed the blackjack table with saliva and invective as she cursed her luck, the cards, and the casino. The banker calmly collected her useless cards and continued dealing the next hand.

Just as Melissa was worrying that a customer might see Earn's outburst, a regular club patron came up to her. He said slyly, "Madam, you said she used to be an air hostess. On which route, the one between Hong Kong and the Macau casinos?"

Having lost all her money, Earn's eyes sparkled when she saw the club patron, and she asked him for a "loan". He was normally quite generous, but was unwilling to give Earn the amount she wanted. She finally accepted HK$500, despite Melissa having taught her never to cut her price in a deal; as once your price falls, so does your reputation. Fearful the customer might change his mind and take his HK$500 elsewhere, Earn was keen to take him upstairs, but her mind was still on her place at the blackjack table. She begged Melissa: "Keep my seat at the table, I'll be back right after the fuck." Melissa recalled that whenever Earn was bought out of the club, she would say to her girls at the nightclub: "Get the mahjong started, I'll be back right after the fuck."

The live-for-today attitude takes many forms. Girls may become prostitutes to clear a lover's debts, or start taking drugs just to demonstrate their love for their junkie boyfriends.

Ah Kuen was a happy-go-lucky romantic girl, who would become excited whenever she heard mainland rocker Cui Jian's *Nothing To My Name* at karaoke. Tai was a long-haired slacker with nothing to recommend him other than his perceived coolness. He and Ah Kuen fell for each other at first sight. Tai sniffed uncut heroin; maintaining his cool façade, he would brag: "This is real." This thrilled Ah Kuen, who began to take drugs to get closer to him.

Before she became addicted, friends tried to persuade her to quit, but she rejected them, saying, "No way! Tai would despise me if I wasn't cool." Her destiny became clear: she had become a prostitute to pay for drugs. She repeatedly insisted she had no regrets about her decision.

Ah Ling had a naturally dour expression. Ironically, she looked better that way, as people found her smile disconcerting. She saw several fortune-tellers who all said she had a hooker's face. Consequently, when she needed money, and didn't wish to fight her fate, she became a prostitute.

After her fourth year in elementary school, Ah Ling had to leave school to take care of her younger brother and sister, who seemed to take this sacrifice for granted. Ah Ling took this badly and became bad-tempered and irritable. To avoid arguments, her brother and sister moved out to live with other family members. Ah Ling felt their desertion added insult to injury and she would visit her brother and sister to berate them over their lack of gratitude or loyalty. Eventually, Ah Ling's family would hang up the phone the moment they heard her voice.

Now she was ostracised, she took her anger out on her neighbour, who was more than a match for Ah Ling. She stood up for herself, and with a piercing voice, she would get the better of Ah Ling in their arguments.

Meanwhile, her boyfriend swindled her out of a year's savings, which she had made from working in a local teahouse. This worsened her temper further and she had a fight with the kitchen workers, during which she offended one of the older members of staff who washed dishes. Subsequently, this individual took her revenge and spat into Ah Ling's soup. When Ah Ling found out about the soup incident, she felt so sick that she went to hospital to have her stomach pumped.

When the hospital doctor told Ah Ling she had brought it on herself and had made a fuss over nothing, she started a fight with the doctor. Taking a taxi home from the hospital, the driver took a longer route than Ah Ling expected, so she started another argument with the driver, shouting at the top of her voice.

Reflecting on her troubles, Ah Ling concluded she was surrounded by devils. It seemed there was never an easy day and she had to be constantly alert for crooks and bullies. Possibly aggravated by stress, she found herself developing thyroid disease. She started to show the typical symptoms of bulging eyes and a swollen neck. The nervous irritability associated with the condition caused her to be increasingly cantankerous at the smallest provocation. Making friends, or maintaining any kind of normal social contact, was virtually impossible for her.

Once, she was late for work and the teahouse manager scolded her. Convinced someone had told him, she spied on her colleagues for the next week to identify the informant. Events such as these would give her sleepless nights, which would make her like a dead fish the next morning. Her tiredness would cause her to muddle orders for tables she was waiting on, which made her suspect someone was tricking her into making mistakes. She constantly muttered to herself, "There are no good people in the world! Living is such a drag! An early death would mean early heaven!"

In the lane behind the teahouse, there was a junkie, Ah Hui, who heard Ah Ling's constant muttering. His comment to her was, "If you are going to die anyway, why not have some fun before you go?" Ah Hui told Ah Ling that after taking drugs, he found the world was not such a bad place. Although Ah Ling was always on guard for crooks, and was naturally suspicious, her defences crumbled for Ah Hui and she fell for him without hesitation. If her new lover said the white powder was a panacea, and he seemed at peace, why not try it? And so it was that after her first fix she too found the world a much, much better place.

Ah Ling's teahouse salary could not pay for her new habit, so she had to prostitute herself at night. When Ah Hui lost his income, Ah Ling had to buy for two. She started in a blowjob house, and then a one-woman brothel, which made easy money but required much patience because of the constant waiting alone for the next customer. When the customers were plentiful, she had no time to take the powder. Just like other prostitutes on drugs, she finally ended up on the street – despite which, since meeting Ah Hui and becoming a prostitute, she had never known sadness. However, she knew the addiction was killing her when she had to hold on in tears while a customer seemed to be screwing her forever, hard and crude. "That lousy fuck, banging like a pile-driver, why couldn't he come and then go!"

Prostitutes all carry their personal baskets of problems. Thinking about their work seems to make them more depressed. If forced to think, they often feel the whole world is indebted to them for doing its dirty work, and are plunged into a self-pitying reverie. Thinking is therefore taboo. More brains, more worries. Freedom from thought equals freedom from problems and cares. The survivors tend to have adopted a policy to "think of nothing". In conversations I've found frequent use of these phrases: right now, this moment, this second, tomorrow I don't care and I don't fucking want to know. Margaret, an older hooker, has a favourite phrase: "The future is in the future, it's none of my business", while 19-year-old Vickie would say, "Dump the lunch box after finishing your lunch, what's there to think about?"

Whether high- or low-priced, male or female, prostitutes seem bad at budgeting their money. In addition to the costs of gambling and gigolos, female prostitutes enjoy spending freely on a daily basis. A few times, I was taken out for midnight snacks, and my host would only decide where to go after getting into a taxi. The taxi would already be in the cross-harbour tunnel heading towards Hong Kong Island, and my host might suddenly decide that the pickled egg and meat porridge in the New Territories was particularly tasty, so the driver would have to make a U-turn. A midnight snack might have a surcharge of a HK$500 taxi fare.

Madam Eiko, the owner of the Japanese-style nightclub, is retired and had a conventional education. She said that when she was a young prostitute she lived without any plan for the future. Her work helped her see through men, leaving her no appetite to be a woman. She felt like she had lost her soul and that her own life mattered little. The resulting numbness left two choices: either give up, or enjoy any stimulus available just to feel something. Based on her 40 years of nightclub experience, Eiko said that most prostitutes have had ugly lives stretching back into childhood.

Squandering money is an external attempt to achieve a momentary flash of pleasure to compensate for an internal emptiness – a dead soul. Despising one's own life easily leads to wild behaviour without limits. Decadence is no big deal. Get high when the wine is fine, be cool, and enjoy the chemistry wherever it can be found; take any chance, any choice, at any time.

Eiko told me that many of her girls had lifestyles based on rational decisions. Most of them were single mothers, forced by circumstance to earn money in the best way they could to fit around their other obligations. They were hardworking, punctual, and respectful to customers. They were thrifty and took good care of their families. Eiko preferred to hire women with children. Maybe they carried more fat, but she would always ask customers to look at their inner beauty.

It seems that there are some prostitutes who lead ordered lives, but I have found it hard to meet them. By their very nature, they have a longer-term view of the future and are concerned for the status and reputation of themselves and their families. They compartmentalise their sex work, and shy away from people not associated with prostitution because they expect to blend seamlessly back into normality at some point in their future.

These 'good' girls are hard to find, but I did manage to meet one genuinely dedicated, hardworking prostitute. Ah Heung's sole purpose in life was to make money, and then more money. She could not even spare time for simple things such as clothes shopping. She had no fun, no friends, no affection, no past, and no future mapped out; work was everything. She couldn't survive a minute without a customer.

When she was bored, she liked to talk to social workers who were the nearest thing she had to friends. Her main point was always, "No customer, no money. Then what can you do?" When she found out that none of the social workers had managed to buy their own apartments, she was startled: "Ah! So you haven't bought an apartment yet. Aren't you scared?"

In the global economy, each trade sector is becoming increasingly organised and regulated. Prostitutes remain unaffected by this trend. They eat when they are hungry, put on clothes when they are cold, gamble when they are bored, and look for love when they are lonely. If a prostitute's lover wants to leave, she will either curse his bones or take fastidious care of him like a precious pet. If he is determined to go, she will fight to the death to keep him. She will cry like a lunatic when hit by sorrow, and if she has to deal with tedious customers she will take it out on a gigolo. If in a particularly nihilistic mood, she will take drugs. This live-for-the-minute approach is hardly compatible with the organisational and administrative procedures used in other industries or in other professions which employ so many workers.

Perhaps living for now is short-sighted; perhaps it is an antidote to the inevitability of mortality. 'Get high and die' is certainly a popular theme in literature and art, but for most of us, the future remains a lottery.

# 13

## MALE PROSTITUTES

The host club industry in Japan and Taiwan enjoyed an expanding market in the 1980s. Prior to the recent sudden growth of host clubs in Hong Kong in the late 1990s, there had been only one such club here. It was opened in the early 1990s by two local male prostitutes who had learned their trade in Taiwan.

This club was located in Repulse Bay to take advantage of the wealthy local women but it managed to survive for only a year on a handful of customers, who were variously old, fat, skinny, ugly, and had bad breath with equally fragrant personalities. The club owners had been prepared to maintain a reserve fund to develop a customer base but the hosts were reluctant to work for no salary, and fierce competition for the few customers caused serious problems.

Striving to be top-class gigolos, the club's hosts had taken loans to buy brand-name clothes and watches. Jealous competition among the heavily-indebted gigolos became so ridiculous that they even blackmailed the customers and their families. There was no control over the blackjack table and a round of drinks could cost HK$35,000. When customers ran out of cash, the house had to take credit cards. The number of high-value transactions caused banks to become suspicious of racketeering and they had the nightclub investigated.

Finally, there was a confrontation between the club and some of the women's jealous husbands, who had four of the most popular gigolos beaten. Another reason for its closure was harsh competition from too many freelance 'gold-digger men' who had entered the business. Although the staff of the Repulse Bay club took a few years' break, they never lost their urge to service women and they finally tapped into an unexpected market of great potential – nightclub hostesses. They became prostitutes for prostitutes.

Host nightclubs may indeed appeal to a certain, very small, minority of liberal middle-class women. However, such women are a rare species in Hong Kong, and are already so spoilt by attention and flirting from male colleagues, bosses and friends that they have no inclination to patronise male prostitutes and are extremely unlikely to visit host clubs. In addition, if they were found in a gigolo house, it would be evidence that they were unable to attract men. Furthermore, visiting a gigolo house would be an expression of their personal interest in sex, and that is an unwritten taboo among these 'liberal-minded' women. Only the sex lives of others are open for comment.

Hong Kong people are more sexually reserved than the Taiwanese. Hong Kong women tend to view their pussy as a means to an end, not as a source of pleasure, and view sex simply for pleasure as a 'business loss'. Therefore, even if sorely tempted by intense curiosity to visit a host club, they would be most unlikely to experiment as a customer as they would still consider the male hosts to be taking advantage of their precious pussy.

Hong Kong is also relatively small, so the chance of running into an acquaintance on the street is high. The few women who might be bold enough to patronise a host club run the risk of being seen, so no matter how frustrated or bored they are, it is safer to stay at home and watch TV.

Men like to be prostitutes to the degree that they have no hesitation in advertising the fact. Male and female prostitutes share the same dream: to meet a powerful, rich partner so that there is no need to struggle, gaining the additional satisfaction that they can survive comfortably on the strength of their personal glamour. A gigolo may dream of mastering his rich lover's affections and of taking command of her wealth, so that he could enjoy money and power ever after. Gigolos reject the idea that their work is a double-win situation – money and sex. They find they have to invest their affection and emotions, and find they are dealing with an increasing number of problematic women.

One gigolo said that when he first had the idea of becoming a male prostitute, his mind was filled with romantic expectations. He was so impressed with the film *Titanic* that he had seen it eight times. He wanted to copy the grace of the hero so that he too could win the favours of a lonely, pretty, high-class girl. A successful gigolo told me that he used to be treated like dirt, but since he became a gigolo, nobody had the nerve to look down on him. If anyone sneered at his prostitution money, he would proffer his wrist and say, "My watch is worth HK$300,000; which part of your body is worth HK$300,000?"

If it really were possible to achieve the double benefit of sex and money, it would help to compensate for the low income. Unfortunately, too few Hong Kong women use gigolos. From 1990 to 2000, Hong Kong newspapers occasionally ran advertisements for male escorts and 'public relations' officers. According to host nightclub owners, a single advertisement would immediately attract several hundred applicants. This raised the bar very high. Anyone who was not handsome, graceful or patient enough, was not sufficiently well groomed, could not make small talk, had no sense of humour or could not sing or dance well enough, would be told to wait at home for further notice. Desperate to be gigolos, many applicants refused to leave their interview, begging for a chance to be a prostitute. One gigolo applied seven times, and another in his forties was so eager to be a gigolo that he was willing to work for three months with no base salary.

Hong Kong gangsters found their profit margins being eroded by amateurs flooding the sex market. Seeing the endless supply of would-be gigolos, Hong Kong gangsters created a scam to make quick money using fake agencies that placed convincing advertisements recruiting gigolos and offering a monthly salary of HK$30,000. The eager applicants came from all walks of life: clerks, transport workers, models, students and married men. The applicants were so keen that they happily paid for highly priced

HIV blood tests at designated clinics, which shared their profits with the agencies, which would later inform the Aids-free applicants there were no customers for them.

Another scam was to demand deposit money from applicants to guarantee the safety and privacy of the rich female customers. Because many applicants believed that once they had business they could make HK$32,000 a night, they would readily incur loans to raise the HK$16,000 deposit. So many men were deceived that the truth was finally realised – the agencies simply could not provide enough customers. The men's desire to become prostitutes vastly outweighed the available female clientele.

Gibbie had been a prostitute for only two years and she had already used several gigolos. However, because the gigolos were not financially desperate, they were unwilling to play the submissive roles requested by Gibbie.

As she could not control her paid-for Hong Kong lovers with money, she went to Shenzhen nightclubs to find male 'PR' officers who might be more grateful for her dollars. Sometimes she found what she wanted; other times she did not. As a consumer, Gibbie felt the gigolos who didn't know how to make her happy did not even deserve her anger; she just stopped seeing them.

Eventually, she found a Shenzhen nightclub singer who charged 1,100RMB for the whole night, and who would lick her all over and give her five orgasms. In effect, each orgasm cost her only 220RMB, while her customers would have to pay HK$1,300 for their orgasms. Gibbie thought this was a good deal and was rather satisfied: "Men play me; I play men; it's fair."

Conventionally, prostitutes use lovers to pass on the disrespect, roughness, contempt and ill treatment they receive from their customers. Paying for a lover is the ultimate cost of being a prostitute. Even though prostitutes' lovers are effectively kept men and are being paid for a service, they usually take the money with no real attempt at offering tenderness or understanding. However, the rapid development of the consumption culture has caught up with prostitutes' kept lovers, who have had to rethink their position as they are increasingly replaced by commercial gigolos, who previously may have been kept lovers themselves.

Prostitutes are realistic enough to see that gigolos are just businessmen underneath, and should adhere to the adage "the customer is supreme". As consumers, women are entitled to enjoy their rights. After finishing their work, they flock into duck houses (host clubs) and leave fat tips to anyone able to make them happy and forget the tediousness of serving customers. This business relationship is settled with no emotional involvement, leaving both parties free of guilt or obligations.

The first duck house aimed at prostitutes was overwhelmed with business from the start; a few other clubs set up and found a similar response. For the convenience of the hostesses, the gigolo houses were located near their nightclubs, with business hours running from midnight till dawn.

Why did nightclub hostesses suddenly develop a taste for gigolos? The attraction is certainly not the price. Hostesses may charge HK$1,500 for each sex deal, while a gigolo's price might be HK$4,000. The answer appears to be that within just a few short years, nightclub hostesses have evolved from social butterflies into sex slaves, who have to accept the five and seven flavour sex package deals every day. The change in market conditions means they have had to accept this, but without any outlet to release their stress and frustrations. Their boyfriends did not present an appropriate target for pent-up stress and self-loathing. The solution that worked best was to offload onto gigolos.

Gigolos, therefore, become shrinks for wounded chickens, making them feel human and able to experience tender feelings again. With hostesses using gigolos in this way, gigolos in turn suffer both physical and emotional exhaustion. This fatigue is their particular occupational hazard, but it allows women who need the warmth to build up the confidence to continue living. Accordingly, if they feel rehumanised and psychologically rejuvenated, prostitutes don't mind paying the price and pumping up gigolos' wallets.

To cater to this need, gigolos have to adjust their professional dreams if they are to serve a chicken clientele. Partly because of the size of their fees, prostitutes will only patronise gigolos when they feel they have reached a mental low point. Gigolos accept that to stay in work they must face a bunch of frayed, ragged, depressed chickens.

One gigolo told me: "As soon as they lay down their asses, those lousy chickens begin to ridicule my farmer's hairstyle and my out-of-date suit. They always make me feel like I'm digging money out of the shit pit."

I once witnessed a hostess walk into a gigolo house and demand time with two gigolos. She then turned into a raving monster and cursed them until exhausted, after which she threw down a wad of notes and left.

Gigolos catering to nightclub hostesses usually don't need a big penis, but they must have a strong stomach. This is because a major part of the job is to play drinking games with the hostesses. They often end up lying drunk in the street at dawn, and then going home to finish throwing up whatever they have left inside. Hostesses like to get gigolos drunk; they like to put down a HK$1,000 note to lure gigolos into a drinking contest, with the best drinker getting the biggest tip. Their favourite treat is to see gigolos totally wasted, so they can verbally abuse them and tell them to imitate a dog barking, or suddenly strike their genitals and then burst into wild laughter at the pain they have caused.

For many gigolos, the worst part is the chickens' insistence on kissing. Although they are mostly pretty young women, gigolos feel sickened by mental images of how the chickens use their mouths for their work.

One Shenzhen gigolo said that most of his customers are Hong Kong chickens who are very hard to please, and making any cash out of them is tough. Gigolos may find they are cursed and beaten if they are unable to keep a permanent erection.

In truth, if a gigolo could exercise his brain a little, he might find himself becoming a champion among his kind. The bottom line is that he is dealing with a woman in need of love like any other, but who blocks her feelings in order to be able to pursue sex work. She uses a gigolo in an attempt to buy back love and human affection. Many gigolos cannot see this simple truth, and think that hostesses have all become sex maniacs who come to them because their customers fail to satisfy their sexual desires. Seasoned gigolos have an idea that they should sell good love and not a good fuck. This means the emphasis is not on a cool appearance or a seductive manner, but the willingness to take on a hooker's love, which is often overpowering.

Once a hooker is in love, it is utter and complete. She will offer her heart and soul, and all her prostitution money. If a man accepts this form of love, he runs the risk of having to supply on-demand attention and affection around the clock. To put it bluntly, prostitutes' use of gigolos is not much different from the drug addiction of traditional hookers.

When my friend Michelle and I finished the 9:30pm movie and left the cinema, the gigolo house was just opening for business. Seeing we were new, the waiter led us into a private room. The public relations manager came to us and said, "You two are so early." He handed us his business card. "My name is Kelvin. At your service any time."

In the top corner of the card was the word "Question" and underneath, in a large circle, "YesterdayYears". The card seemed to suggest an enquiry of the past. Kelvin saw me looking at the design of the card and seemed excited: "Many people only come to their senses when they are older. They have no balls to face joy when they are young, wasting their youth for nothing while blaming others for giving up their innocence."

"So, you are demanding customers question their past?" The philosophical element intrigued me. Kelvin said: "I've been here for eight years, and you are the first person to appreciate the house name." The ice was broken and the general atmosphere seemed pleasant enough, so I gave up the detective approach, and Michelle relaxed.

Kelvin's appearance was agreeable rather than stunning, but he had a friendly manner. With a dark suit and a silk tie, he sounded well educated and his manner reminded me of a decent bank clerk. The diamond watch on his left wrist indicated his sub-cultural taste. He had a provocative sense of humour likely to whet people's appetite for fun. His frequent pats on our shoulders and laps did not offend us. It reminded the beautiful Michelle of her late teenage years when she was surrounded by flirting admirers.

After briefing us of the prices for services, Kelvin asked what type of gigolos we wanted. Seeing we were embarrassed, he said: "It's gigolos that we sell here. If you don't give clear instructions, I can't make good recommendations, and you'll buy pain." Michelle replied: "I don't want anyone too young." In no time, he brought in two male PRs in their late twenties. Michael sat beside Michelle, and Elton sat next to me.

These gigolos were subtle, not flirtatious like Kelvin, and talked with common sense and good taste. They were quite professional and attentive, feeding us with peeled grapes. I didn't enjoy this, but Elton said that this princess-serving style is a favourite of customers from Southeast Asia. Michael said that many women dared not seek fun in Hong Kong, so they would go to Thailand, but they could not have real fun because of the language barrier. Even though Thai gigolos could not engage in small talk, they could offer first-class hand-feeding dinner services to cater to female Hong Kong customers.

It seems that many women customers like to be hand-fed. I was told that even 18- and 19-year-olds, blessed with money falling from the sky, would come in groups demanding two gigolos each to provide wining and dining services.

Kelvin walked in. "Are you playing hand-guessing games?" Michael and Elton instantly responded: "No way! They are too delicate to play such games!" Elton told me, "Almost all my customers want to play hand-guessing games." Kelvin sat down, and said: "You are special guests." Then he signalled the two gigolos to leave and asked if we wanted them replaced, saying he had some good stock. We said, "We don't want to change, now we've got to know each other." Michael and Elton came back to the room, and this time Kelvin didn't leave. He seemed to enjoy chatting with us.

Kelvin had been one of the owners of the Repulse Bay host nightclub that created a stir in the early 1990s. As a young stud in his prime he could make half a million dollars a night. Every day he would put on a different suit worth HK$30,000-40,000, and he was a regular patron of nightclubs. He would demand a dozen or even 20 hostesses to fulfil his lust, and the bill was usually over HK$200,000, which was only a tiny slice of his colossal income.

Before starting as a gigolo in Hong Kong, Kelvin had worked for four months in a host nightclub in Taiwan, making some money and discovering his talent for the profession. The club owner didn't want to lose him and offered him a share in the business, but Kelvin wanted to open his own club in Hong Kong to continue his extravagant lifestyle. Before starting up in business, he chose to extend his apprenticeship and went to work in various host nightclubs in Japan and America.

Returning to Hong Kong, he chose a discreet location in Repulse Bay to protect the female customers' privacy. At the beginning, it attracted a few rich women, but Hong Kong is small and soon everyone was familiar with each other and the club lost its sense of mystery. The familiarity meant the popular gigolos were quickly identified and would be bought out in long-term deals. The other customers did not want the leftover gigolos, even if there was no charge. Kelvin had to scale down the business and move to Causeway Bay. Throughout peaks and troughs in the general economy, which have caused prostitutes of both sexes to suffer, Kelvin's club has managed to make slow progress.

Reflecting on his career as a prostitute, Kelvin's eyes showed intense flashes of love and hate, totally at odds with his apparently carefree personality. After pausing for a few seconds, he summed up: "There isn't a simple conclusion. Sweet, bitter, sour, spicy, just think of all the words in your vocabulary. I've gained so much, lived like a king, and I've lost even more. I've seen right through human nature. Life has no fun for me any more."

During his days in Repulse Bay, frustrated women in their fifties would come to Kelvin. They had no sense of humour, couldn't sing, and couldn't dance; they just had complaints about being life's victims. He treated them in the same way a responsible psychiatrist would treat his patients; he would just listen, taking them for a drive and letting them air their buried grievances. Once people are given the chance to whine, they go on forever. The frustration of these women loomed like a mountain. Professional psychiatrists would have a tough job with these women, and would deserve every penny of their fees.

Once their anger had been vented, Kelvin would begin to feed their sexual starvation. Sex always led to jealousy. His love-all style would naturally incur disputes, even violence, and he had to use political strategies to stay out of trouble. He was often the subject of an auction: when Mrs A wanted to buy him out, Mrs B would offer a higher price, and then Mrs C would chip in with an even higher bid. These wives would bargain down their husbands' parking fees, but when it came to Kelvin, they were eager to shower him with money like it was confetti. He didn't want to be auctioned, so he signed long-term contracts with four women, to run consecutively.

Kelvin never concealed his profession and no one despised him for what he did. Many men wanted to study his tactics and learn how to conquer women. He considered himself a terrific fuck and was always willing to teach his customers. Once a customer's sexual technique was improved, her husband or lover would fill her purse, and the grateful customer would, in turn, fill Kelvin's wallet.

A gigolo's job is more complex than that of a female prostitute, who tends to have a simple sex relationship with her men. Gigolos have to establish more of a personal relationship and connect with the soul. Kelvin asked: "Why do shrinks have to see other shrinks to keep their mental balance? Simply because entering someone's soul is not a pleasant thing, and entering the soul of a patient is like visiting hell!"

Prostitution for Kelvin is like a doctor/patient relationship. The patient has a lifelong chronic condition, which cannot be cured until death. During treatment, the doctor is developing his own chronic illness, so he has to see other doctors for his own worsening condition. Kelvin made money from women and spent money on other women. He made a fortune from being a prostitute, while spending it on other prostitutes.

Feeling numb was the root cause of his pain. He felt he had experienced a whole life in eight years. He had made a lot of money, and squandered it. He had cheated the love of others, and others had deceived him. Somebody had cut her wrists for him and he had swallowed sleeping pills for someone else. He had been humiliated and had stolen the dignity of others. He was still young, but his passion for life was long dead. Nothing hurt more than feeling nothing. He wanted to climb out of the shit pit, but he enjoyed the taste.

Two years ago, I accompanied a sociologist to Kelvin's club, but he was not there. It was said that after being bought out by a well-respected Macau gangster madam for a few months, he had put on weight and now did not want to be seen by anyone. More recently, I took a film director to the gigolo club to collect material, and he was still not there. Apparently, his habit of showing off his luxury watch and expensive car had infuriated some desperately impoverished gigolos, who nearly crippled him in a beating.

Elton was handsome, with simple dress and a plastic watch, and not a shred of evidence of the gigolo sub-culture. He was a hotel clerk and had decided to join the profession after a year of unemployment. Half a year's work had given him all the experiences he bargained for. He cooked himself a special stew every day to maintain his stamina. Each night, he would go through the same routine and play the drinking game with women. He had to guess hard to win; if he lost, the alcohol would punish him. Usually he would be drunk by 2:00am, but 4:00am is the rush hour period in the gigolo club. To keep going he would splash ice water on his face, make himself throw up, and go back for more of the drinking game. By the time he finished in the morning, he would feel like death warmed up. Sometimes, a kind customer would take him home; sometimes he would take a cab home. In the back seat of the cab, he might drift off in a dreamlike trance and end up at the terminal taxi rank.

Elton had worked hard, and ended up with some good customers, who neither whined nor complained, nor wanted to drink. They just needed his shoulder, and like sacks of soft sand, they would lean against his chest and weep until daybreak. Some customers were not so good tempered. The pitiful ones might turn into ferocious harridans, making him suffer, telling him to act like a monkey or a dog. Working in this profession, Elton had learned to forgive the unhappy ones. He saw them as unlucky ulcers filled with anger and frustration. His job was to soothe away the pus.

Talking to me, Elton was attentive and caring. Seeing me not talking, he asked, "Have I bored you?" He wanted to tell jokes to make women happy. He did not enjoy being teased by co-workers that he was a lady-killer. What he wanted was to be a killer with successful hostesses, who were generous with tips and gifts. However, these prostitutes scorned him for not being wild enough. He felt he had staked his life on the drinking game for nothing.

Elton's attentiveness had allowed him to nurture several regular patrons who were second wives. One would come every night and demand his company. She would sit there for a couple of hours, with no fuss and no drinking games, just leaning her head quietly on his shoulder. Seeing her off each time, Elton would be amazed, touching his shoulder and wondering how it could sell for thousands of dollars every night.

Another second wife offered to buy him out for a satisfactory price, but she would constantly sigh and whine, saying, "I'm so lonely! What's living for anyway? Come and die with me!" The woman's dejection scared Elton, who did not understand how more experienced gigolos could raise families of their own while maintaining the favour of several frustrated and depressed women.

One older gigolo was simultaneously serving a celebrity's first and second wives. For a year, these two women had no idea they were patronising the same gigolo, and the celebrity had no idea what was happening while he was finding time for yet more women.

Elton was waiting for his fortunes to change. He hoped that one day his birthday party would be as magnificent as Kelvin's. He said with envy: "That night, Kelvin's customers bought him ten thousand fresh roses. The entire house was buried in roses: the entrance, all over the ceiling, the stairs, the walls, in the restrooms, everywhere was roses."

People in this profession believe in retribution. Their job is to make women happy, and yet the unhappy women simply demand too much, and the gigolos have no panacea to satisfy their demands. The women seeking thrills usually end up even sadder. Unhappiness comes from a mindset that thinks happiness can be bought. Husbands ignore their women, who squander their husbands' money on buying attention from others. Using gigolos is taking revenge on men.

Elton planned to work for two years. He just hoped he could avoid the worst of the women's anger, so that they would not humiliate him in public or have him killed.

Elton stressed his reluctance to offer sex services. He repeatedly said: "It's hard to imagine that someone could sell that for easy cash." For Elton, dignity was more important than money. He hoped that in his two years in prostitution, he would meet a high-class lady like the girl in *Titanic*. She would love him and be willing to give up her luxurious life; he would love her in return and spend his life keeping her happy.

Two years ago, I ran into Elton on the street with a woman shopping for clothes. He was decked out like a typical duck star: pomaded hair shining in the sunlight, black shirt, red suit, and a wrist-watch decorated with diamonds the size of pigeon's eggs.

# 14

# Ah Dong and Gee Choi

In 2002, two gigolo club-owners offered the following story. The events may be apocryphal, happening in different places with different people. Despite this note of scepticism, the story illustrates the way informants see their own world of male prostitution, and provides an insight into the love-hate relationship between female and male prostitutes in Hong Kong.

Ho Feitong owned a duck house, which is Hong Kong slang for a club providing male hosts, or gigolos, for female clients. He was once a gigolo himself and was quite used to living the high life when money was plentiful, then losing it all gambling, only to earn it and lose it all over again. After 12 years, he had a bagful of tricks to entice female customers. Unfortunately, his charm dwindled as his waistline spread, so his only option to stay in the business was to open a brothel and train new gigolos. He was surprised to find that both customers and gigolos had evolved so much that his personal experience and bagful of tricks no longer counted for much.

He placed an advertisement for male 'public relations' personnel, which is a well-understood euphemism. On the first day, he was surprised to see so many applicants queuing up for the walk-in interview, all smartly dressed in business suits. One hopeful, in a greenish-yellow suit, looked like a banana to Ho Feitong, who had a personal dislike of bananas, real or otherwise. "Try an orange suit next time," he suggested. Another began his interview by boasting of over 100 one-night stands. Ho Feitong took a closer look and admitted to himself that the interviewee had a certain suave arrogance, which reminded him of Rudolph Valentino. However, he would never let a one-night stand master ruin his business, so he responded: "Being a male PR has nothing to do with one-night stands. I am running a business to satisfy customers, not enter a competition."

Another candidate simply bragged that he was a terrific fuck. "Enough, enough!" Ho Feitong said, "How about you ask a woman, any woman, to lay down a pile of money in front of you and then you see if you can work on her without taking an aphrodisiac. Even if you are hung like a horse and you know how to press the right buttons, can you do it to order, time after time? My next advertisement will make it clear: Super fucks don't bother."

Ah Dong was a handsome candidate. He heard the applicant before him rejected as follows: "You've dressed so casually for this interview, how could I send you out to meet a customer?" Hearing this, and considering his own shabby clothing and the well-dressed candidates around him, he felt depressed and slipped away. He borrowed money from loan sharks to buy top-class brand-name menswear. He enjoyed the flattering service of the shop assistants, which for the first time in his life made him feel dignified. He was so thrilled by the experience that he borrowed even more from the loan sharks for another shopping spree.

Armed with his new clothes, Ah Dong returned for an interview. He saw a well-mannered man begging Ho Feitong: "I've answered so many ads that only tried to swindle money from me, it's not easy for me to meet a serious businessman like you. It's fate that we should meet like this. Can you just give me two months' probation? I don't ask for a base salary, and I'm ready to learn and work hard." Ho Feitong was not impressed: "You've watched too many gigolo movies; you think you know too much already. How can I train you?"

Ah Dong was next. He swaggered like a model in front of Ho Feitong, who saw the selling points in his look, his body, and the quality of his clothes. He asked Ah Dong to start work later that day.

After only a month, Ah Dong had become a star host and the regular female clients fought to buy him full-time. Ah Dong preferred patrons who came from a simple background. Although they could be rough talking, they were direct, and it was easy to find out what they wanted to keep them happy. They were often generous in their appreciation. Ah Dong didn't like to serve mistresses; he found their unresolved romantic lives made them time-consuming clients and he could not maintain his attention.

He was a poor singer and dancer, but was particularly good at playing Taiwan-style hand-guessing games. Pleasing lady customers came easily to Ah Dong. He felt the trick was to carefully and constantly observe their facial expressions to know what was wanted, and in return he found he was often showered with gifts.

Once, Ah Dong invited a VIP customer to the Regent Hotel for dinner. He prepared a wad of HK$50 bills in his pocket, from which he deftly peeled tips from the hotel entrance all the way to the French restaurant on the third floor. This stylish extravagance impressed the lady customer, who felt flattered at the respect and deference shown to her by the hotel staff. After the meal, Ah Dong received a watch worth HK$60,000.

Hostesses finishing work were not so difficult to please, but had their own ways of being troublesome. They would often flock in at three in the morning, as if they had synchronised their watches. They would come in groups, all demanding his instant company. Pleasing one meant neglecting another.

Whether the girls had been serving customers themselves or not, once they came to the gigolo house, they had to be treated with ultimate respect. These wild customers could be extremely generous, but they would die to save face. A few regular groups would demand Ah Dong's company every night, with no concessions to each other. Catering to one group would give him problems from the other. Women in the losing group would make snide comments: his hair was looking greasy or his eyes were too small. Once these bitching mouths started, they would never shut up. Ah Dong became the whipping boy for all the women's repressed feelings which had built up during their work as hostesses.

Ah Dong could only put on a polite smile and swallow the insults. His job demanded him to be courteous and civil to all, so he was obliged to move among the groups, only to be bullied again by others. No one properly understood where the girls' rage came from, but it continued nonetheless. The comments and insults tore at his heart and soul without mercy: his face was too broad, his voice was shrill like a cockerel's, he had no dress sense.

Under this constant barrage, Ah Dong's confidence dwindled, so much so that he had no heart to participate in the Hong Kong gigolo contest. This lost him a rare opportunity to gain peer recognition as a consummate professional. He began to hate the hostess clients, but for the time being, their generosity kept him working.

Another new gigolo, Ah Tsuo, had an appearance and mannerisms that often caused him to be derided by the hostess customers for reminding them of their own clients. Each time the manager sent him out, customers would have him replaced, saying, "He looks so much like my customers. I'm paying the bill now, and you want me to pay for him? If he stays another minute, I'll charge him my hourly rate!" Seeing Ah Tsuo's problems with the better customers, Ah Dong kept him busy with his headache customers – the unhappy mistresses.

Although Ah Dong had made a very successful gigolo career for himself, he still had a weakness for decorating himself with expensive brand-name goods, which meant he would still use loan sharks for money to feed his habit. He would put himself in debt for a diamond ring, an exclusive watch, the latest mobile phone, a tailored suit or crocodile-skin shoes. Whenever he showed off his gigolo accomplishments in front of friends, he would do so with great pride. He would often treat his family and friends to feasts, and if anyone despised him for being a gigolo, he'd fire back: "My shoes are worth 9,000 bucks, each time I do my hair, it's 1,000 bucks, and my lighter is 18 carat gold and covered in diamonds. Show me something you have that's worth as much!"

Nightclubs often organise 'Champion Hostess' contests. Once, there was a competition for the 'Most Bought-Out Hostess'.

Gee Choi, a young, pretty, sexy, slutty-looking hostess, would win all the titles every month. Securing the title of 'Most Bought-Out Hostess' was a piece of cake. Riding high with confidence and self-satisfaction, it was a shock for Gee Choi and the other winners when an army of northern girls seemed to descend on Hong Kong nightclubs. Not only did they have lean, curvaceous figures, they also bragged they could harness *chi kung* to give customers extra pleasure. Many nightclubs saw an opportunity for lower costs and new blood. Local hostesses were suspended, and gazed on with green eyes as their customers were snatched away by the northern invaders.

Gee Choi couldn't take the humiliation of seeing her customers taken away by northerners, and pleaded with her manager for help. He told her that the nightclub had been incorporated, and the operation was now controlled from elsewhere. He advised that the best plan was to compete head-on. If she wanted to save face, she should look for something new to offer. Perhaps she should study customers' fantasies submitted to *Call Girl Directory* and work out new sex tricks to beat the fad for *chi kung* sex.

Gee Choi used her bought-out hours to practise and develop her 'multiple sex games'. To defend her 'Champion Hostess' title, she was prepared to offer new services. Soon, several of her techniques became popular and her business boomed. By the end of the month, she was elected one of the top ten most bought-out hostesses. The effort had severely stressed Gee Choi, and her temper became very highly strung. Her madam talked her into going to a gigolo house to offload.

Meanwhile, pressed by creditors, Ah Dong was becoming desperate for money and was telling his regular customers: "Whatever you need, just name it, I will do anything to make you happy."

His hostess customers understood perfectly well that Ah Dong made the offer not for their pleasure but for their money. They wanted to find his lowest price and asked him to state it clearly. Ah Dong needed money so badly that he agreed. He gave his minimum price and went along with the customers' prerequisite of a three-orgasm guarantee. Under this pressure, his performance suffered during sex. It reached the stage where his regular customers sometimes had him replaced, even after he had used Viagra.

After two weeks' hard, non-stop sex work, Ah Dong finally cleared his debts. This relief was spoiled by the realisation that his reputation as a lover was ruined at the nightclub, and he was now a figure of fun during the drinking games. Some ill-intentioned regular customers would buy him out to lend him to other clubs, just to let others see the notorious "limp noodle, greedy, lousy fuck".

Gee Choi came to Ah Dong's club. The gigolos would drink when she told them to, and imitate bed screams on demand. Gee Choi had a good time, but was outraged when the bill arrived. "You fucking gigolo! How dare you charge me four times the price I charge my customers!" She cursed endlessly, but came back every night, with the same fury and insults at the size of the bill.

Her pleasure appeared to come from seeing the gigolos suffer, for which she accepted paying four times her own price. Behind her back, gigolos gave her the nickname "lousy chicken", and nobody liked serving her.

Seeing Ah Dong had lost all his regular patrons, Ho Feitong sent him to serve Gee Choi. Thus began Ah Dong's journey into hell. Every night, he had to tolerate abuse and humiliation to make a living, because yet again he was being squeezed hard by creditors.

One day, Gee Choi ridiculed his hairstyle in front of others. The biggest taboo for gigolos is criticism of their appearance. Burning for revenge, Ah Dong went to Gee Choi's club, and asked for her company. He then took the opportunity to dismiss her body as worthless in front of the madam, violating the same taboo in return. After this humiliation, Gee Choi went to Ah Dong's club after finishing work. She homed in on Ah Dong and openly and loudly made fun of his body and lack of physical charms. One good turn deserved another. They had become addicted to each other, and both now had to work a little harder to earn more to pay for the pleasure of the verbal abuse.

The duck house had a new customer, Dana, who came with a private chauffeur. She was no longer young and she did not look like a prostitute, so Ho Feitong sent out Ah Tsuo, who specialised in catering to mistresses. Dana liked to occupy a private room and play innocent romantic games with gigolos. Sometimes, she would bring in a butterfly, set it free in the room, and ask Ah Tsuo to chase it with her. Sometimes, she'd bring in a big sack and demand Ah Tsuo be tied up inside it. When he was tied up inside the sack, he was to leave the private room and leap around in the club just to scare people. Sometimes, she brought costumes and dressed Ah Tsuo as a female, just to show him to others in the club.

Ah Tsuo accepted these freakish games, and for no other reason than his patient forbearance, he had won the sympathy of several of top-class hostess patrons, who promoted him in their estimation from 'lady killer' to 'hostess killer'.

Ho Feitong often resorted to his own experiences to lecture gigolos on how to cater to customers. His tricks, however, were developed in another age among rich women, and were hardly relevant to hooker customers. Consequently, none of the gigolos would listen to him. Seeing a dead fish like Ah Tsuo make a fortune, Ho Feitong encouraged Ah Dong to serve Dana. He used his past glories to teach Ah Dong how to work on lonely women, how to satisfy their fetish for gigolos, and how to make them squander their money.

Ah Dong followed his boss's tricks to develop a romantic approach, and he hit the bull's-eye. Dana declared that she was indeed born into a rich society family, but she had always been unhappy. When she was young, she tried to commit suicide for love. Although she survived, she lost the will to live and turned into a vegetable. Her father spent a huge sum for a year of specialist treatment in Switzerland, after which she seemed to improve. However, she later made another suicide attempt for another lover. This time, her psychosis was diagnosed as more severe than had been thought, and it cost her father another fortune for treatment in America. She recovered, but her youth was gone. She was now buying herself lost romance.

Ah Dong felt he was too naive to handle this, so he gave a complete version of the complicated story to his boss, seeking his advice. Ho Feitong immediately congratulated Ah Dong: "You have finally met your fortune. For the sake of money, you have to love her, at least for a year or so, even if you can't love her for a whole lifetime."

He instructed Ah Dong: "Never charge her for sex, but make sure you fuck her real good to make her addicted to you. By then, you needn't worry about her money; demand whatever you like." Following this advice, Ah Dong took her to bed, applied himself diligently, and fell asleep after the job. He woke up to find his expensive watch and bracelet missing.

A few days later, Dana came to the nightclub as if nothing had happened. Ah Dong confronted her and demanded the return of his property. Dana calmly denied everything, saying: "Look at my car and private chauffeur. Why would I need to steal your shit?" Ho Feitong believed Dana and asked Ah Dong to back down and not offend a customer. He was planning to bait Dana himself.

Ah Dong had lost his treasured possessions and his face, and to a regular patron. He was so mad and disheartened that he felt he needed to find Gee Choi to purge his feelings of anger and resentment. The nightclub madam told him that Gee Choi was not in the mood for work that night, and was not there. Disappointed, Ah Dong returned to work, only to find Gee Choi waiting impatiently for him.

She opened fire the moment she saw Ah Dong, who detected in her abuse that she was angry because a client had taken her cash and jewellery. This was too much for Ah Dong, who suddenly lost control and cried out: "I beg you please, my sister, just for now, let me go! I've really had enough tonight! My things have been stolen by a regular customer, and it was a customer I've been working on with my heart and soul." Gee Choi relaxed and called for the bill. As she walked out past Ah Dong, she stuffed her remaining cash into his pocket.

The next day Ah Dong went to call on Gee Choi. Instead of teasing her as usual, he just sat there quietly for the whole evening. He called for the bill and as he left her, he handed her a wad of cash with the words: "I hope this will make up for what you lost." Holding the money and watching him leave, tears welled up in her eyes.

Ah Dong and Gee Choi continued to see each other professionally, but now in a different way. They would sit quietly with each other, resting their heads on each other's shoulders. Paying for each other's time was very costly, so they worked as hard as ever to make more money. Gee Choi still had many regular customers, and Ah Dong, now having a high-profile patron like Gee Choi, became popular again in the duck house, but for a peculiar reason. Gee Choi's rivals sometimes came to patronise him out of spite, just to get back at her.

Meanwhile, Dana became Ho Feitong's regular customer. Dana told him that her father had passed away, and taking advantage of this low point in her life, Ho Feitong seized the opportunity to be more attentive and supportive in order to take total command of her emotions. She would not allow him out of her sight for a moment. Ho Feitong was waiting patiently to make his move on her money, when she asked him first to lend her HK$950,000 to pay inheritance tax.

"Only after paying the inheritance tax can I inherit my father's wealth and sell his property," she said. "I've made a rough calculation; it's worth 200 million dollars, enough for the rest of my days. Once I have the money, I'll repay you ten times over. If I can't pay the inheritance tax, I'll be dead."

Ho Feitong did his own calculations. If he did not invest the HK$950,000 to pay the inheritance tax, not only would he lose the huge return, but also all the energy he had spent on her, and his face would be lost in front of the other gigolos. He sold his car, his watch, and his investments to raise the money. When she was given the money, she took her time and wanted to have sex with him. Thinking of the HK$950,000 blood money in Dana's handbag excited Ho Feitong and spurred him on. After an unusually energetic performance, he sighed in amazement: "I haven't had sex as good as that in a very long time." Dana replied: "Men only fuck well when they've paid."

Then, Dana simply vanished, leaving Ho Feitong searching for her like a maniac. He would lose his temper at the slightest provocation, even cursing women in front of customers. The gigolos feared he would scare off trade and persuaded him to take it out on cheap street hookers, which he did.

In Sham Shui Po, he spotted a street hooker who looked exactly like Dana. He wanted to buy her and give her a hard time. The clock hotels in that part of town charge for rooms in periods of 15 minutes, and it is the hookers who have to pay for the room. In order to fix the cost, they have to finish business within the first 15 minutes. To save time, they only partially undress. This habit makes them feel that taking off all their clothes is unnatural or even shameful.

The Dana look-alike rejected his demand to take off all her clothes, so he paid another HK$100 to get his way and have her naked. She gave in for the money but, standing naked in the customer's loathsome gaze, she felt so humiliated that she returned the money just to put her dress back on. She turned around to dress. This coyness excited Ho Feitong, who threw down even more money, and before she could put the dress back on, he ordered her to turn around naked once again.

From that point, he became a regular visitor to Sham Shui Po. Although a frequent patron, he never touched the hookers' bodies; he just looked at them naked, and masturbated. Seeing that he was a good customer, the women decided not charge him extra.

His temper improved a little, but his heart would still ache whenever he thought about the emptiness he felt. Sometimes he would sing karaoke alone in his duck house, and always failed to hold back his tears when he came to the line *'Return my love'*.

Hostess clients sympathised with him, and this gave Ho Feitong a lot of business. The club manager saw the demand, and charged double for his time, which gave him enormous pride. Although he no longer had his youth, it reminded him of how much he enjoyed his gigolo career.

One day, Ho Feitong saw Ah Dong and Gee Choi walking into a shop selling wedding gowns. That night, he asked Ah Dong: "Why hasn't

Gee Choi been in for so long?" Ah Dong mumbled, "She's fed up with it all."

"Maybe she's developed a new fetish, for wedding pictures," said Ho Feitong. "Your business is so poor these days, if someone buys you out for a few years of marriage, I won't stop you from quitting."

Ah Dong replied, "We are not playing at weddings. We are getting married."

"For real? Then I won't stop you," said Ho Feitong.

"After the wedding, I'd like to continue working, to be a really good gigolo," Ah Dong said. "Gee Choi wants to change profession, and I need to support her. So can you help me and loan me two months' salary to pay for the wedding?"

Ho Feitong refused at once. "You don't have many customers now, and you'll have even fewer after you get married. I won't lend you the money, because you will never be able to pay it back."

Ah Dong tried again: "With your loan, I can get married. If I get married, Gee Choi can do phone sex, and if she can do phone sex, she can help you retrieve that HK$950,000." Ho Feitong was puzzled. "What has my HK$950,000 got to do with your wife's phone sex business?"

"When Gee Choi applied to the phone sex company, she saw that old fox Dana was the owner of the firm. The two of us, Gee Choi and me, will play games with the old bag. So, if you want your money back, let's work out a plan."

This insider's story holds considerable value in highlighting areas worthy of further social and cultural studies. It illustrates a linear progression within the sex industry: a capital transfer from well-heeled men to high-priced prostitutes, then from lavish prostitutes to gigolos, then to cheap street hookers, and finally to drug dealers. During the process, the waste – or anger – generated along the way is excreted through orderly internal channels, without any government resources being required to clean up this community pollution.

# 15

## JOYFUL CHICKEN

All the hookers I have met are hopeless at organising their lives, and seem doomed to suffer financial and emotional problems. I was about to give up the search for a happy, confident whore like Norma Jean Almodovar, when I met Dou Dou.

Dou Dou never liked to study. At school, she would daydream, and spend all her time in class gazing into the middle distance. She was happy to join the noisy after-school crowd and do whatever took her fancy. Despite appearances, she was smart, and even though her textbooks remained untouched, she still managed to pass her graduation exams. On finishing high school, she itched to do something rebellious, but could find nothing to capture her imagination. To pass the time while she decided what to do, she became a secretary in a Japanese trading company. One year of typing made her feel she was wasting her life and she became determined to find something else.

She was nearly twenty years old when she was first solicited. She was pleased she had been noticed and was wildly happy from the illicit thrill. The customer subconsciously switched roles with her: lighting her cigarette and filling her teacup. He eventually asked, good-naturedly, "Am I hooking you or are you hooking me?"

This was going to be her trademark, the confusion of roles between server and served. Customers enjoyed their time with her and would laugh freely; they may not remember what the drink was called, but they would never forget Dou Dou's name. Customers would often feel relaxed enough to indulge in childish horseplay; maybe they would put their necktie around their forehead, imitate a cockerel crowing, or even try to perform somersaults like the Monkey King. They felt they could leave only when Dou Dou had been entertained in return.

For more reserved customers, she would not let them go until they could recite "Dou Dou is a happy hostess" in Mandarin, Fujian dialect, English and Japanese. Dou Dou joined the business for a simple reason. It was fun.

Most of the girls were desperate deadbeats and worked in the business to keep from starving. These were the girls who liked to stress they were forced into this grim situation; victims who, underneath, were pure at heart. Dou Dou never fell for that. In front of other girls, she would ask the customer: "Are their poor cunts lined with gold?" She would mock other girls' methods: "Stop playing the pitiful whore; even if you could give the cliché new life, your pussy is still the same."

The girls who knew Dou Dou were embarrassed by her unapologetic confidence. They could only fall back on well-worn platitudes: "it's all I can do", "even the poor have pride", "vanity kills", "I have a family to raise", "it's just to clear my debts", "I have no choice". Dou Dou wouldn't put up with any of that, declaring: "You would all be better off if you didn't waste your money on gigolos. And if you keep slandering me because I enjoy my work, and calling me unnatural and depraved, I'll fuck you to death."

Dou Dou never lacked money and other girls often borrowed from her. For the sake of the money, and knowing the views of their banker, the indebted girls dared not play up their misfortunes.

Dou Dou had a short memory. Ten minutes after a fight she would be flirting and joking again. Her speciality was to dress up customers in women's clothes, bras, wigs and heavy make-up. She would make them play the sissy, with rewards of sweet kisses. For hostesses, the worst possible failure is being unable to heat up the atmosphere and then placing the blame on customers. This produces bad feelings in themselves and is unfair to the customer. Gradually, all the sisters accepted Dou

Dou's happy-go-lucky attitude and they liked to spend time with her, having good fun and wild times.

Some hostesses have great ambitions, and obsess about business or financial miracles. Dou Dou thought little of these idiots with impossible dreams who had no understanding of either the jungle of the real world or their own capabilities. Regularly, girls with very little money would leave to open shops, only to report to the madam after a year to start work again.

In Dou Dou's eyes, prostitution was the best trade in the world. It involved messing around at work with friends while meeting people, learning new things all the time, and making quick money. All it took was briefly opening one's legs. Even the customers who banged hard like a mule pulling a carriage could be made to finish quickly with a few moans and caresses, and an encouraging word or two. As far as she could see, her pussy didn't suffer; even after a tough session, all that was ever needed was a brief rest afterwards. Entrepreneurship? Start a business and buy trouble? Change profession? Crazy!

Dou Dou had no financial problems and was completely free to pick her customers at will. During the first year, she was filled with curiosity to see how different men fuck, so she would take anyone without flu or who did not look too dirty. She was straightforward and she didn't play coy. She was considerate, but was not a soft touch. Virile customers would be rewarded with extra time, while impotent ones were encouraged to just quit.

Numerous sex partners brought her to the conclusion that sex was merely a boring game, in which there was no such thing as true ecstasy. Pornographic films and literature were full of shit, dangling the honey pot of sexual promise in front of foolish, easily duped losers who had no real chance. She was not to be taken in, for she had met too many and knew too much.

Although she no longer fancied sex, she still took all customers. This was not because she liked money, but because she liked people, and through sex, she could maintain her relationship with them. No matter what trouble she had, the minute she was with a customer, all her worries were gone. Her customers were her friends.

A few years later, Dou Dou discovered, through her career, that men did not really find good women that attractive. She felt she was a good woman and could thus never win a man's passionate interest. She slowly came to dislike this part of the male character.

Dou Dou was always true to her feelings and fearlessly expressed her interest in all types of men. She would take any customers and accept any deal without a trace of self-conceit. In the sex industry, nobody appreciated the quiet, sincere, hardworking attitude that she had learned in her first office job. It seemed to be the pretentious, childish, cold type that customers favoured. Although madams had to treat these girls with kid gloves, they realised their commercial value and offered them to customers like golden pineapples. It was so unfair.

In order to fulfil her ambition to be a top-class prostitute, she copied the style of the mean, tricky hostesses. She put on airs and graces with customers, started fights with procurers, and only went back to a hotel after repeated invitations. She ordered the most expensive foods and, when offered a gift, picked the most expensive item. Soon, she transformed herself into an arrogant hostess of taste and style. She had believed that saving money for others was at least good for her conscience, if not an actual virtue. She had been too dumb, customers were only with her because they had the money to burn; they were protected by a wife at home with a tight grip on the household expenses. It was not her concern to economise for the customer.

She was the wild flower on the wrong side of the fence. Her job was to be a bad woman, wicked and coquettish. If hostesses were just like housewives, why would men visit them?

Mastering this approach, she unexpectedly found men saying things to her like "I would carve your name on my bones", "I hate you because I love you too much", "I have never wanted a woman as much as this" and "You are my ultimate woman".

Dou Dou was touched, but conflicted. She tried to be a good prostitute and follow the unwritten professional code that one should never fight for another's husband. One of her newly found worshippers was Ken. He was a not very good-looking bachelor who was the manager of his father's jewellery factory, where he was on call around the clock. He was a patient man, and would play 24 rounds of mahjong without complaint, letting her take the bet if she won and reimbursing her when she lost.

Ken became serious about Dou Dou, saying he wanted to marry her and telling her to quit her work. She refused, saying she enjoyed her job and would keep on working as long as she found it fun. As a compromise, he asked her not to strike sex deals, and she said: "Relax, I'm frigid." He was not satisfied with this, so while she was at work he went to her nightclub and found her with a customer. He called another girl to join him in the next booth and they started to play hand-guessing games, which is accepted to be foreplay and a signal that things will go further.

When she realised what was happening, jealousy turned the slightly built Dou Dou into a ferocious tiger and she stormed into the next booth, tearing apart the kissing couple and knocking bottles and glasses onto the floor. She grabbed the girl's hair in one hand, and gave Ken's face a mighty slap with the other.

After this fight, Dou Dou lost both her love and her face. She was heartbroken and shed tears whenever she sang romantic karaoke love songs.

Determined not to give in, she vowed to win Ken back and told him she would stop being his professional lover, and hoped they could marry. She waited for his calls for days, around the clock. Ken's passion was gone together with his patience. His tolerance of her behaviour was dwindling. Within a few minutes of meeting her, he was picking out her faults. Night after night, Ken went window-shopping in nightclub lobbies and waiting rooms, maxing out his credit cards one after the other.

Ken tried to work out with Dou Dou how much he had spent on her. Dou Dou drew on her savings to pay him back. Then, he disappeared. For days, Dou Dou looked for him everywhere. She was devastated when she finally came across Ken picking out an expensive wrist-watch as a gift for another hostess. Dou Dou kicked off her high heels in disgust and threw them at the couple.

Working in a new nightclub, the depressed Dou Dou gave the madam a hard time finding her a customer fond of sad stories. When she was bored, she played hand-guessing games with the bartender so loudly that the madam would lose her patience and would send Dou Dou to serve any customer just to keep her quiet. Once with customers, Dou Dou found her happiness and she soon built up a regular clientele.

This time, Dou Dou was more calculating in order to make sure she avoided emotional complications. From among her customers she carefully selected a married man to be her lover, and two more customers as backup lovers. She would insist on making the same requests of all three lovers just to observe their different reactions. This was the perfect game for her. Nothing gave her more fun than the study of men.

Being a Gemini, her right brain warned her not to get emotionally involved in love games, but her left brain just wouldn't listen, and she gave in. She demanded Mr A divorce his wife for her, and he simply disappeared. Then she asked Mr B to leave his other women; he did so but found replacements. Fortunately, she still had C who would do anything to please her.

Mr C was a bore, babbling at her constantly to quit. Hard-won experience caused her right brain to advise caution, but her left brain told her to wash away her make-up and be his full-time lover.

For a few months, she devoted herself to studying men who would dump their families to become her full-time lovers. She discovered that a man who would abandon his family for you was worth nothing, even if he was a free gift! The cohabitation with Mr C did not go well. He reminded her daily of his sacrifices and demanded she do this and do that. To repay his sacrifices, she ran the household on a tight budget. Now that Dou Dou the exciting lover had changed into a surrogate housewife, Mr C lost interest and didn't return home every night. Running out of money, he lured a cheap girl from an unlicensed nightclub back to the house. Dou Dou had driven away his wife; now it was her turn to be replaced. She could not forgive herself for letting this happen, but this painful lesson was her graduation from a trying course: 'Knowing Men'. Dou Dou came to realise that men who use prostitutes do not deserve a woman's loyalty.

'Don't treat men too well' is an adage well known by women, but rarely followed, for most women have a limited choice of men at hand.

Dou Dou returned to the nightclub with a better understanding of male psychology. She entertained and controlled customers freely, and she found the confidence from her hard-gained knowledge allowed her to enjoy the work again. Being a hostess needs no formal education, but Dou Dou had gone to school and she used her ability to solve problems to design a clever timetable.

For the seven days of the week, she had seven keys made to her apartment and gave one to each of seven regular customers, who felt obliged to contribute to her house rent. Collecting seven rental payments each month was not an easy task, since she had to invent neat lies to ensure that each man, during his designated days, used his key like the master of the house.

The seven men all believed that she had a troublesome sister and a stubborn mother who interfered too much in her private relationships, worried she would become involved with a married man. Consequently, there was a risk they might show up and visit her at any moment. This meant there should never be any trace of a man to be found in the house. If Monday's man wanted to reschedule to Wednesday, she first had to check that her sister was leaving Hong Kong for the mainland on Wednesday. If the Thursday man wanted to come on Saturday, she would have to confirm that her mother would be out playing mahjong all night long.

Maintaining this juggling act required a very good memory, which Dou Dou had. She could make instant justifications to cover any slip of the tongue, then immediately lodge the revised story into her mental filing system in case of repercussions.

For a year, she received her rent from the seven unwitting men without problems. However, six of them were putting her under pressure to give up hostess work, and two of the six wanted her to start a small business to keep busy. She had no interest in business, so she excused herself for not having the necessary skills. Three men asked her to be a full-time concubine. In principle, that would be nothing new, for she had been the simultaneous mistress of seven men. Eventually, one man came to accept her reluctance to leave her job, and asked her to be a madam instead a hostess.

Dou Dou knew that being a madam was not as easy or as much fun as being a hostess, but at least she could stay in the business. She promised she would stop being a hostess. On becoming a madam, she had to think about the company's profit all the time. She had to deal with the tough girls, and find work for the less popular girls, while generally encouraging customers to spend money. She came to regret being influenced by men to give up her favourite work. Every time she saw one of her girls bought out, she felt a pang of nostalgia.

Two men handed back their keys in the second year and left her for good, so she found substitutes for Thursday and Saturday. Soon after, Monday and Tuesday left as well. She could find no other men to fit into her timetable, so she accepted the vacancies and bided her time for fear of spoiling the whole arrangement.

Living on men was devouring her youth, and the 30-year-old Dou Dou knew only too well that her prime would not last forever. Her expenditure was not great as she hardly gambled on horse racing, and played some mahjong only occasionally. Her liabilities were her sisters, who always had tearful stories to tell of their endless debts. At that stage, her savings were just not enough to guarantee a sound retirement.

The Asian financial crisis hit, and drove customers away one by one. Sometimes, the club would not receive a single customer for the whole evening. As the madam, she was responsible for promoting and maintaining custom. The poor level of business led to unpleasant confrontations with the club boss. She hated the job of madam, but was too old to be a hostess again. Besides, the men paying her rent were all strongly opposed to her prostituting herself. Her days were not as easy and fun as when she was a hostess, yet she still kept playing hand-guessing games, singing karaoke, talking dirty, juggling her time among boyfriends, and occasionally finding lovers for Monday and Tuesday.

Dou Dou wanted neither a baby nor marriage. She hated planning for the future. Sometimes she looked into her crystal ball and told herself she would be a madam for the next ten years. After 20 years she would be 50, and what would she do then? Dou Dou decided she might open a bar; she could still play hand-guessing games, sing, talk dirty, and serve beer.

I was to see Dou Dou again four years later in her club. She was in an explosive, irrational mood, standing akimbo on a low table ranting at a girl for nothing more than poorly applied eyeliner.

It seems her delicate timetable had failed. She had been suspicious that her latest lover at the time had a sexually transmitted disease, so to ensure the safety of her other lovers, she proposed the use of condoms. The men said, in their own ways, that they maintained their relationships with her for exclusive sex. If they were to use condoms, they could use hookers, and save money. Dou Dou feared that she might become infected, and so she had lost four of her private, rent-paying lovers. This is what had caused this tough, shrewd woman to lose her temper over nothing more than eye make-up.

# 16

## POCKET-MONEY SEX

Japanese youngsters exchanging sex for pocket money is now a common phenomenon. Their aim is not to make money as such, but to supplement their parental allowances in order to afford brand-name clothing and accessories. These young people are adamant they are not prostitutes. Their reasoning is that they do not rely on the activity to survive, and they can choose what to do, and when, usually when they want a new handbag or designer clothing. Trading youthful bodies for trinkets and pocket money is not limited to Japan.

In Malaysia, there is the 'bohsia' girl, roughly translated as 'silent' or 'mouth shut' girl. The conservative establishment now uses the term 'bohsia' to describe various forms of youthful activity that it finds unacceptable. Latterly, it has become an umbrella term that includes the activities of young males.

The particular 'bohsia' incarnation that has caused most consternation is the original stereotype of a young girl from a comfortable background spending her time in and around large shopping malls and standing at strategic locations to attract the attention of older men cruising by, either on large expensive motorcycles or in luxury cars. Neither the man nor the girl says anything as she accepts a ride, and the implicit deal is done. Neither, of course, does the girl say anything to her unsuspecting family.

Not to be left out, Singapore has the notorious 'SPG', or sarong party girl, who has become a national anti-icon. Historically, the cliché is that local girls, dressed in sarongs, would wait outside the long-gone British army bases on the evening of the soldiers' payday. The soldiers could choose one of the waiting girls on their way into town.

Today, 'SPG' is used to describe, often pejoratively, the stereotype of a young girl who is typically taller, more tanned, and less generously clothed than her Singaporean sisters. She appears to harbour a particular interest in Caucasian men and seems little concerned if they are significantly older. She perceives the benefits to be access to a more liberal lifestyle, a partner with a larger wallet and penis, and a potential ticket out of Singapore.

A generally similar phenomenon, more akin to the Japanese experience, exists in wealthy, middle-class Hong Kong society. If parents in an affluent society can afford to educate their children, and provide them with a comfortable lifestyle, why do 15- and 16-year-olds still prostitute themselves for extra spending money? Teen hookers in Japan and Hong Kong had the following explanations when questioned by social researchers:

"My allowance can't buy me Chanel stuff."

"Schoolmates all have the latest mobile phone, how can I not have one?"

"My boyfriend likes expensive gifts, I can't give him stuff too shabby."

"My cunt is no longer a virgin, but it's still worth 3,000 bucks, so what am I saving it for?"

"The best is to meet the weak old guys, they can't really fuck, and I still make cash."

"I wanted a new yellow motorbike, but my old man gave me an old black one, so I had to go and work in a duck house and make the money in my own way."

"I was walking on the street, a man came up and asked about my price, I said I was on my period, so he wanted to pay me 2,000 bucks just for going to dinner with him. I insisted on 3,000 and he agreed."

These youngsters make no effort to conceal their prostitution; instead, they brag about their prices. Young girls do it to avoid the shame of going to school without a brand-name handbag. Teenaged boys enjoy enormous pride and status if they find work in a duck house, and enjoy showing off gifts received from women.

A situation like this cannot be dismissed with the phrase: "Each generation gets worse!" In a materialistic culture created by adults, youngsters suffer huge pressure to consume. They feel inadequate if they do not have the same things enjoyed by their peers. Parents chide them, "You are so vain! How can you have luxury before you have hardship!" Their prostitution is a silent protest against the adult world. Young people pursue the same pleasures as adults. Their attitude is: "You have shaped our aspirations, we are following your lead, so we know what's 'good' and what's 'bad'."

When May was 13, she decided she was terribly bored and offered herself two options: either die or live for the sake of pleasure. Even if she chose to die, she wanted to indulge herself beforehand. Accordingly, with nothing to lose, she would fall in love with a spendthrift, happy-go-lucky boy, then fall out of love when he declared himself broke. Sometimes this could all happen in one day.

Although disappointed with her one-day adventures, she counted herself lucky as she could still have sex, and make money, so she became a whore at the age of 14. After two years, she declared herself so experienced that her customers could not find better.

Having been in such demand, she felt there were so many interesting, generous men ready to spend money on her. She decided the best way to take advantage of her abilities would be to stop working on the street and work in a nightclub. May was deadly envious of older girls who were able to work as hostesses. However, at only 16 and a half, no first-class nightclub dared recruit her. She yearned for her 18th birthday, for which she was planning a lavish party in a grand nightclub, where she could invite her many regular patrons.

Vickie quit school when she was 13 and made friends with a gang of streetwise boys. Together, they started peddling pirated compact discs.

Within a year, she was a mini-tycoon with a monthly income of at least HK$30,000. When she was 15, the disc business was at its peak, and she was making HK$45,000 a month.

Before she reached 16, the government authorities began a general clampdown on the pirated disc business and she had to close her little shop. She had spent all her money and had to find another job. Although intelligent and pretty, she could only find poorly paid jobs, which she thought was a huge waste of her youth. Once, when she was offered HK$7,000 a month as a shop assistant, she simply turned around and walked away without saying a word.

After looking for work for two months, Vickie had managed to find nothing to suit her. All she could find was work as a karaoke hostess, singing along with customers. She did not earn as much as she was used to, but could make it pay if she let customers touch her. She went with a group of prostitutes to Japan on a working holiday, making money interspersed with frantic bouts of shopping. Returning to Hong Kong, she reminisced fondly about her Japanese customers and their taste for unusual sex. With the few Japanese sentences she had learned, she sounded like an old hand at the business.

Vickie decided: "Japanese customers seem to like freaky sex, but they are fun and I'm going back there."


A hundred years ago, women had negligible political and economic rights, which effectively made them the weaker sex. Men considered women irrational, meddlesome, and prone to crying. Female emancipation during the 20th century has proven those ideas wrong. The fruits of the feminist movement have included different age attitudes and politics. As an area of study by liberal and modernist sociologists, 'age politics' may provide rational interpretations of teenage prostitution.

Age politics identifies the most powerful as the married, middle-aged middle classes, with established careers and steady incomes. The elderly have less power because they generally rely on others for support, including welfare or state pensions. Children, having no obvious power, are viewed as the future of their society and are invested with attention and resources. Young people on the verge of full adulthood benefit from their innate vigour and enjoy many of the benefits of adult life.

The remaining, weakest group, comprises teenagers from 13 to 18 years old. They are leaving the world of children, both physically and psychologically, and coming face to face with adult supervision and control. They suffer additionally from an 'immature teen mentality' which age politics identifies as a prejudice held by adults.

At a community seminar in Hong Kong, a female sociology professor presented various theories to argue that prostitution is not a sin, and that it should be accepted and supported instead of reviled. She then elaborated on the physical and mental maturity of teens in modern society. The audience was receptive to her ideas, and some parents present supported her view that the "don't argue, I know what's best for you" approach with children should be avoided in order not to strangle their potential.

The professor also contended that teens indulge in pornography because adults have mystified sex. Preventing youngsters from seeing anything with a sexual content simply provokes their curiosity. Even the older members of the audience, who one might otherwise have expected to be conservative, agreed with this assertion.

Finally, the professor touched on the most sensitive issue: sexual activity. She thought it not an issue that youngsters decided to become part-time prostitutes. It was like working at McDonald's; they were just learning to support themselves. Indeed, to work for McDonald's was to be exploited by a multinational conglomerate while prostitution represented self-employment, earning rewards proportional to the effort. Students studying overseas would commonly engage in temporary prostitution to support themselves.

The parents present were much less comfortable with these views. The professor went on to explain that exploitation of child prostitutes is simply a rumour disseminated by anti-prostitution activists. Real exploitation occurs when fast food outlets take advantage of the cheap labour of youngsters. Prostitution also provides direct encounters with people, which is a good way to learn about life, she explained. These last comments were too much for the parents, and one mother bursting with anger shouted: "Maybe your ideas work in theory, but do you have children? Would you let them be prostitutes?"

When Kam To was in her third year at junior high school, none of her classmates were using mobile phones, but many of them were sporting brand-name clothes. With an 'easy come, easy go' attitude towards money, they enjoyed a profligate lifestyle as seen in *True Youth*, a local soap opera. They would hang out all day long having a good time, singing karaoke, and enjoying front-row concert tickets to see their favourite artists.

Kam To longed for the soap opera-defined luxury of *True Youth*. She felt her own youth was slipping away minute by minute, spent eating, watching TV, and engaging in daily trivia. When she was 11, her parents would send her away with HK$5 for candy. At 13, this rose to HK$10 and now, at 15, they gave her HK$20. A line from a popular song taken from a Cantonese-language film goes: *'You remain a child forever in your parents' eyes.'* To Kam To, such parents were simply insulting their children's intelligence.

Kam To decided to take care of her financial problems by singing karaoke in a Mong Kok club, where she met a couple of schoolmates. Working in pairs tripled the friends' courage, and everybody had a good time. After a few months, Kam To's hymen was auctioned to the highest bidder. She exchanged her virginity for a Cartier wrist-watch.

Progressively armour-plated by brand names, the fledgling chickens and ducks now found themselves in an armour-plated patrol wagon after a raid by the vice squad. Her confused parents were desperate to save face while bailing her out from the police station, asking, "We are in good financial shape, so how could she possibly be a karaoke girl? She must have hooked up with the wrong people."

When they got home, her father threatened her: "If you do that again, we'll send you to a reformatory." Her mother interrogated her friends and accomplices. Her busy parents' attention was soon diverted by their daily working lives, and Kam To escaped any real punishment. Soon afterwards, her half-brother came home and had a huge fight with their father. She took the opportunity of this distraction to find work in another karaoke bar.

Kam To was a classic beauty by Chinese standards. She was taller than average, with clear, pale skin and perfect, uniform doll-like features. When she met Ah On at her new place of employment she was dripping with jewellery. The attraction was instant and powerful. At only 21, Ah On and his partners had a company wholesaling children's clothes, which was a front for their real business of smuggling cigarettes. Having a monthly income of HK$30,000 to HK$40,000, he was a spendthrift. He took taxis everywhere for transport and constantly dined out. He had a weakness for expensive dishes such as abalone soup. His coiffure was by celebrity stylists and he bought whatever was currently fashionable and took his eye. He enjoyed inviting friends to luxury hotels to play cards, and constantly gave gifts and money to Kam To.

Kam To loved this lavish lifestyle as it catered to her youthful notions of luxury and status. The money-burning naturally attracted fair-weather friends, who made it even harder for the extravagant couple to save anything.

Years later, Kam To, who was never any good at keeping track of her spending, was shocked to realise that in just six months of prodigal living she had spent every last penny she had, and this had effectively mortgaged her freedom for the rest of her life.

Ah On's cigarette smuggling was detected by the police and his shop was sealed. He was arrested, interrogated and prosecuted. All evidence proved it was Ah On alone running the business. All the criminal charges fell upon Ah On who was required to make good all the company's debts.

Ah On was no better at keeping track of money than Kam To. He had borrowed from loan sharks to cover his squandering and he owed

HK$150,000. Behind bars, there was no way he could repay the money. The creditors came after Kam To for repayment, saying she had played her part in the reckless spending. Fundamentally decent, Kam To never liked to argue over debts and was always prepared to settle things amicably.

Out of loyalty to Ah On, she became preoccupied with how to clear the various debts, regardless of whether she was legally obliged to do so. She sold all her valuables and emptied her bank account. It was then that two banks started to take action to collect payment for her credit card spending. Ah On had applied for two credit cards in her name, using fake documents. The credit limits had been exceeded very quickly. She now owed the banks another HK$150,000.

The answer was easy! With her alluring looks and slim figure, she could get a two-year contract as a PR ('public relations') lady in a nightclub, paid in advance, to clear the debt. Her joy at striking a two-year prostitution deal was dashed when she found she was cursed with a mean-spirited mama-san who thought Kam To was devious and low-class. Kam To punched in late and knocked off early, and took her problems out on the customers, who repeatedly had her replaced.

At the beginning, her lack of success was indeed her own fault. With Ah On in prison, she was in no mood to serve customers and had no energy or desire to please. When her spirits improved, she felt she was capable of becoming a star PR. However, by this time the mama-san had already developed a prejudice against her, making Kam To the last choice in the nightclub. With no good customers, and no bought-out work time, Kam To knew she wouldn't make any real money during her two-year contract. She realised it would be a waste of her good looks, her lithe figure, and her youth.

Kam To was acquainted with a mama-san at another nightclub, who occasionally called to give her part-time work. She soon developed some regular customers, with more bought-out work time. Kam To would pretend to be sick, only going through the motions at her first job, saving as much time as possible for her moonlighting.

This arrangement lasted for only a few months. Just as she was beginning to make a little cash, her employer found out. The second job violated Article 1 of her two-year employment contract. Her excuses were not accepted and her employer fired her immediately, while simultaneously imposing a fine resulting from the contract violation. The fine was three times her initial advance. She now owed HK$450,000, which was put in the hands of professional debt collectors designated by the nightclub.

Kam To had worked so hard, all for nothing! The new debt hung over her like a huge black cloud. The interest payments were climbing and the collectors were increasing their level of threatening behaviour day by day. She was so desperate she would now take any customers. Despite her desperation, she could not manage to reduce her daily expenditure. Ah On had spoiled her so badly that she just couldn't wear cheap clothes, use local hairdressers or give up playing mahjong.

She had a sister who had made a fortune on the stock market, had no debts, and owned a fancy car. Kam To thought she could do the same if only she had some initial capital. Intoxicated with enthusiasm, but remembering her previous experiences, she approached ten moneylenders. She took her time and selected what appeared to be the least aggressive finance company, which required only one guarantor's signature. This would normally have been easy enough were she still working in a nightclub. Typically, the mama-san would be the first to volunteer to be guarantor, as it would increase her control. The once-bitten, twice-shy Kam To chose a more amenable guarantor: her sister.

Although the two sisters made cautious plans and consulted several advisors, luck was not with them. The stock market remorselessly absorbed their funds. The more she lost, the more Kam To became scared. Her increasingly desperate investments led to a new debt of HK$700,000, which she shared with her sister. By this time, her monthly interest payments alone amounted to HK$100,000.

Kam To was charging HK$1,500-1,800 each time she opened her legs. In a good week, she would have seven clients, but if business was bad, she would only make a couple of deals. Added to payment on an hourly basis for her time, this would give her a monthly income of approximately

HK$70,000, which meant she could not afford to lose when she played mahjong. Despite the ever-present mountain of debt, she still could not curb her extravagant tastes in hairdressing, dining out, and nightlife. Paradoxically, it was only through these luxuries that she could distract herself from the reality of her monstrous debt.

Inbetween the mahjong and her other extravagances, she would be face to face with cold reality and the demon debt collectors, who seemed determined to hunt her down till she dropped dead. How was she to remove this burden? She tried pleading with her family. Her brother had maxed out four credit cards, and the family house was under siege by creditors.

Her father was caught in a complicated triangle of debt, and for inexplicable reasons he became involved in legal disputes and ended up taking on a further debt of two million dollars. He ran away to escape the liabilities, deserting Kam To's mother, who became so paranoid and confused in fighting off the creditors that she would even mistake her daughter for a creditor when they met.

How could she rid herself of this huge millstone? Kam To knew she could sell her pussy, her fairy hole, but the market was in recession. Even if she managed to secure two deals every night and saved hard, she could only keep pace with the rocketing interest. She liked to daydream, wishing some rich man would come along to pay off all her debts. According to her logic of natural attraction, it shouldn't have been too difficult to bait a millionaire with her remarkable good looks; yet, with eyes beaming like searchlights, she could not find a single millionaire no matter how hard she tried.

Learning of her debts, customers who were professionals would be stunned, as if they had met an extra-terrestrial, saying, "My income is less than your monthly interest repayments!" If she was lucky, a businessman might leave a tip to cover two days' interest, then vanish. Her older colleagues told her that customers liked to help unfortunate prostitutes as it flattered their vanity as saviours and demonstrated their innate goodness, as well as increasing their karmic scores in the reincarnation stakes.

Despite wealthy clients' tips, she wondered why she couldn't come across the one single hero she needed. As her hope evaporated, she became panic-stricken. She started to daydream about picking up a 'big brother', someone who could help her with his underworld influence and connections. So she would home in on tough-looking men wearing gold neck chains and open collars. However, these big brothers only wanted to get her to bed for one-night stands, paying as they went, with no emotional investment at all.

Her next daydream led her to a fung shui master, who agreed cash on delivery for results. After several worthless attempts, she dumped him and turned to another mystic, who she paid in advance. Despite this, her debts kept on mounting.

Ah On was released from prison before finishing his sentence. He had been bored to death in his cell and dreamt of luxury, but the first thing on his list was to avoid any future debt. He felt under great pressure and out of desperation decided to sell narcotics to make quick money. Kam To was comforted to have him at her side; it felt like family. Her pleasure was cut short by her sister, who came to press Ah On to pay the debts Kam To had incurred speculating on the stock market.

Ah On went drug trafficking, Kam To went whoring, and their debts kept rising. They became smarter at avoiding their creditors who, in turn, learnt they had to be on the ball in order to track down and confront the impecunious pair. It was like living in hell; they found their situation had become intolerable. Ah On observed the carefree attitude of his junkie customers, who often seemed to be away with the fairies. He gave in and started to buy heroin in larger quantities, for both his wholesale dealing and for himself. He too decided to let himself be carried away by the white powder.

Seeing the change in Ah On, Kam To also took to narcotics and together they enjoyed a short, blind happiness. When the cash for heroin ran out, the withdrawal symptoms left them drawn and ragged, devastating their looks. Even the demon creditors stayed away from them.

Kam To's employer realised what was happening and stopped her from prostituting herself in the lobby of his nightclub. To try to deal with the combined problems of debt and heroin addiction, she started working in a small unlicensed brothel in Mong Kok. Cold turkey made her stammer and tremble, and she would have to make excuses and slip away for a fix. Her appetite for heroin meant she did not survive the brothel for more than a year.

Ah On rented a floor of an old building and opened a one-woman brothel for Kam To. With no other backers or staff, Ah On was also the all-purpose manager and bouncer, and had to deal with customers if they became nasty. Within half a year, they were kicked onto the street for owing rent. A little while later, Ah On was caught harbouring drugs. He was found guilty and sent to prison again. With Ah On gone, the only option left for Kam To was to be a street hooker.

The first time, she tried to charge a little more, telling the customer she was very young for a street hooker: "I'm only 27, that must be worth 400 bucks." The customer replied: "So what? A street hooker goes for a street price."

Her drug addiction was so acute that she needed a fix every three hours. The addiction finally changed her lavish habits. Now, she sheepishly handed every cent she made over to drug dealers. Her hair was greasy and lank, and her clothes grubby and unkempt. She was starting to smell rank from lack of hygiene.

No matter how hard she tried, she could not save enough for the drugs she needed. This was the time of the Asian financial crisis in the late 1990s, which put a severe brake on the Hong Kong economy. Customers were now out of work and she might spend all day on the street without making a single deal. The heroin clock was ticking. What was she to do? Desperate, she would blatantly approach passers-by with a simple offer: "400 bucks, you can fuck my ass."

Since then, I have lost touch with Kam To. The street girls say that she spends more days behind bars than on the street. She has been frequently arrested for harbouring drugs or seducing others to conduct immoral acts.

When found guilty, she would put up a fierce fight, not from the fear of going to prison but of going through the hell of withdrawal symptoms. It wasn't food and other simple luxuries she missed, but heroin. On her release from prison, she would first hook a few customers on the street, then meet with the white powder – her fair-weather friend.

# 17

## WHO WANTS A REVOLUTION?

Prostitutes are a marginalised, disadvantaged group suffering similar social discrimination to that once experienced by homosexuals. Under the influence of human rights movements, mainstream society is now more accepting of homosexuals.

A lesbian acquaintance from a wealthy background said: "Under the heterosexual regime, we were suppressed by mainstream society, and we had to fight for our rights and dignity. Prostitutes may feel a similar repression but they have the choice to change profession. They far outnumber homosexuals, and hookers have always been abused and even murdered, yet they still don't want to come out of their closet to stand up for their own rights. Ultimately, they are a willingly marginalised group."

This is a specious position, as much of the social changes in the acceptance of homosexuality derive from the efforts of homosexuals already holding positions of influence in the arts, media, professions, and even government. Prostitutes, however, have no such pre-existing network.

Now democratically elected to Hong Kong's Legislative Council, Leung Kwok-hung (better known as 'Long Hair') has taken part in many street protests, defending the rights of the disadvantaged poor. He has extensively studied Marxist works and has developed his debating methods from years of political struggle.

I asked him for his argument in support of prostitutes' rights. His automatic response was one of grandiose Marxist rhetoric involving oppression of the workers, which would lead inevitably to the glorious overthrow of their exploiters, at which point prostitutes would be finally emancipated.

I had heard all this before and had to stop him.

"Hey, slow down a little bit! Could you just pretend for two minutes that you are not a knee-jerk Marxist? Come at it from a different angle. Who holds the real power? Does the situation not change because it suits certain interests for it not to? Let's hear anything but the theory of exploitation."

"Save your words! I'll never give up Marxism, but you may just have to rethink your prostitute rights!" said the maddened Long Hair, who seemed to take it personally, as if his political credentials were threatened.

Not able to accept this stubborn dogmatism, I started a heated argument with him. Long Hair is well known for his grand style of oratory in defence of workers' rights. His view was: "Workers sell labour, prostitutes sell sex. It's the same thing, but they belong to different social groups. Prostitutes are a typically marginalised disadvantaged group with no motivation to push forward a revolution of their own."

It was too bad he was born in the wrong era. Standing on his soapbox at the beginning of the 20th century, he could have drawn an audience on almost any city street corner. Now, a century later, the vintage of his politics was showing. The only supporters of his views seemed to be a handful of ageing, opportunistic prostitutes whose income was undoubtedly dwindling. Following their professional instincts, they would have jumped onto any bandwagon for whatever they could extract from it. In this case, it was Long Hair's Marxist bandwagon that happened to be passing.

Hong Kong's political groups, social activists and even feminists follow the conventional model of liberation politics. Like earnest missionaries, they believe in the search for the ultimate truth, to solve all the problems in the world. As an anthropologist put it: "Politicians, revolutionaries and social activists have a problem fetish. Without problems they'd be unemployed, so they create big issues out of petty matters."

Long Hair clarified his position. "Listen to me, anyone who supports capitalist free trade has no right to look down on prostitution. This damn free trade is the hooker spirit. There's no logical difference!"

Who is not exploited in a fast-paced capitalist society? Who doesn't sell something of themselves for money? Scholars sell thoughts, stars sell faces, athletes sell physical performance, singers sell voices, workers sell labour; doctors sell diagnoses, lawyers sell legal knowledge. Which profession is not commoditised? So why is it so unacceptable to trade sex for money?

Should we make a grand gesture and reject our commercialised society, and return to the Stone Age? It would be a wasted sacrifice. Abolishing prostitution is perhaps harder than giving up our much-loved mobile phones, washing machines, cosmetics and brand-name handbags.

Assuming there is nothing wrong with prostitution as an established commercial activity, validated by longevity, we need to finally resolve the issue of prostitutes' rights so that everyone can conduct their profession without disapproval. Are glad-to-be-gay homosexuals more righteous than prostitutes who have chosen not to start their own revolution? Is sex for money any less acceptable than sex without any possibility of procreation? What might prostitutes themselves say?

"A revolution? Are you telling us to expose ourselves in the media? You motherfucker! You nosy sisters, go onto the roof and count your pubic hair [Cantonese slang meaning "don't bother me"]! Just leave us alone. After business, we'll smoke marijuana and play mahjong, and then pick more customers. We've got no time for bullshit chicken rights or duck rights. That rights shit could swamp us with northern girls, which will just fuck up the market. Customers already taunt us, saying that as soon as they walk into a dance hall on the mainland they are surrounded by a dozen northern girls who only charge 60RMB for a half-hour blowjob. That's scary. Give us a break! Stop the rescue crap! Hong Kong's chicken farms and duck ranches aren't that bad. We like the shady style of business. We are free to join or quit the profession, to charge according to the customers and the market, to put on a thousand faces, and maybe even become big stars in the entertainment industry. Maybe we could meet a good guy and get married. If we make enough money, we might start a business. If the business fails, we can always go back to prostitution.

"Maybe we don't have legal protection, but what would Hong Kong be like if prostitution was decriminalised? All the streets would be lined with migrant hookers. Maybe we would be forced to work in a red-light zone. Customers and hookers alike prefer the discreet hustle. In a controlled red-light district everybody would be labelled either a hooker or a John. How could we bargain? How could customers enjoy the chase if it was all so organised? Are we to be doomed to work like battery chickens? None of the high-priced hookers want to fight for prostitute rights."

My lesbian acquaintance may smugly claim that prostitutes are willingly self-marginalised, but she is right for the wrong reasons. The revolutionary Long Hair is reluctant to accept that prostitutes represent a special case, and would never support such a crusade even if he had resources to spare. A prostitute rights movement can only be driven from street level. As the upmarket call girls, escorts and club workers have said: street hookers are a floating group of northern girls fighting for business, here today, gone tomorrow – unlikely warriors in a workers' revolution.

Northern girls are outside the legally visible labour force. The moment they walk the street they violate immigration law, which makes them unable to mount a formal legal effort to fight for their rights. Members of this transient group enter Hong Kong on short-term permits and work to such tight schedules they may not even have time to change their clothes before they return home. They are not the most likely candidates to mobilise themselves for a socio-political struggle. The drug-addicted hookers are no more likely to act, as any energy they have is likely to be focused on finding the next fix.

Taiwan is cited as a Chinese society that has effectively organised and licensed prostitution. In 1949, the Kuomintang brought many mainland soldiers to Taiwan. To comfort the soldiers, organised prostitution was permitted. Licensed women had a mark tattooed on their foreheads. This lifelong indicator of prostitution made it very difficult to change profession. Although unlicensed hookers were everywhere, licensed women were still able to bring in a monthly income of NT$200,000, thanks to a selling point of better hygiene.

President Chen Shui-bian was formerly mayor of Taipei. To canvass political support from middle-class women, he joined a moral crusade to advocate "family priority", to oppose "money for sex", to save "hookers who sell sex for money", and to root out "gangsters' exploitation". Since the beginning of 1998, the authorities have conducted a large-scale anti-vice campaign which has devastated the sex industry. Large numbers of prostitutes and gigolos have changed profession, and licensed prostitution was finally abolished in 2001. Female supporters of Chen Shui-bian's moral stance gave him their votes, helping him to consolidate his political position. Licensed hookers were crushed, and in order to survive, they were willing to join hands with any possible source of support. They continued fighting for their livelihood for several years. The strength of the prostitute rights movement in Taiwan is a direct result of Chen Shui-bian's repression.

Naive intellectuals with no knowledge of prostitution, including myself at one point, are fascinated by the notion of the happy hooker.

Purple Vine is an organisation with the aim of promoting the idea of the happy hooker throughout Hong Kong society. The Purple Vine vision is well known among Hong Kong academics. This is because the two ex-hooker members of Purple Vine lecture everywhere they can find a receptive audience, preaching the message that despite rotten working conditions, prostitutes enjoy orgasms during their work, and that sex services provide a positive social function.

Purple Vine seems to have deterred their potential membership which, after several years of operation, still comprises the same handful of superannuated hookers. However, this 'prostitutes' union' has been rather more successful in attracting local intellectuals as members. When I was scratching around for interview subjects I approached Purple Vine, the secretary-general of which was no more helpful than to suggest I go and find girls on the street. It was then that I wondered just whose interests Purple Vine actually served.

Hong Kong prostitutes like to operate off the radar. The more Purple Vine seeks attention and makes headlines, the less attractive it becomes to its potential members. The same principle applied when the Hong Kong Health Department set up clinics in hospitals for prostitutes on the basis that there would be no waiting and no queuing. This initiative required patients to inform the clinics that they were prostitutes, and consequently, the clinics have served almost no patients at all. Even now, after years of existence, Purple Vine can still only muster eight or nine masked individuals for a street protest, the majority of whom are more likely to be intellectuals than sex workers. How can such an organisation claim to represent its claimed constituency?

Voluntary groups cannot survive on theory alone, and most of their income is derived from donations. Philanthropists generally determine their donations according to the group's scope of operation. Since northern girls are equal in number to local girls, Purple Vine has expanded its remit to include them. However, northern girls could not care less about dignity or prostitute rights. Neither do they fear running into friends or family members on Hong Kong streets. In view of the enmity between Hong Kong girls and northern girls, whose rights is Purple Vine fighting for?

In contrast, the Blue Bird organisation fully understands prostitutes' dislike of help provided by voluntary groups with agendas. Accordingly, they maintain a low profile with no grand ambitions for a prostitutes' revolution. They simply offer advice, guidance and limited social support. After years of operation, they finally extended their range of services from local street hookers to include Philippine and Thai prostitute communities. These foreign prostitutes simply leave Hong Kong after earning enough, with no interest in taking part in a social revolution.

Blue Bird continues to play the low-key social worker while Purple Vine continues to push its concept of sex workers' rights under the noses of academia and the government's public policy research sector. Both voluntary groups find they can only target the more visible prostitutes, i.e. the less sophisticated streetwalkers. Caring for this group requires particular sensitivity: too much enthusiasm will deter, while inadequate attention will be met with disdain.

Street girls have no patience to reason with society for equality of rights – they appear more driven by simple greed, which can't be satisfied by a fair society. They would prefer to invest their energy in a wealthy customer with money to burn, or make a wild gamble to win enough to quit the profession. They are tired and cynical. Want to turn them into happy chickens? Simple. A little heroin will do.

The movement to abolish prostitution originates from the notion of the 'miserable prostitute'. Activists holding this view do not want to accept the fact that women join the profession of their own will, and they try to rescue these sad, fallen women. Liberal feminism, however, attempts to replace this 'wretched hooker' concept with the establishment of equal human rights and dignity.

It is the happy chicken theory which affirms that sex work is a free, professional choice. This is similar to the assumption of rational choice in neoclassical economics, which presumes that every individual can equally and fully access information to make a rational decision, in order to maximise his or her self-interest. To function, this argument assumes that everyone is free from economic, cultural, political and social restrictions, which is far from the case.

The influx of foreign sex workers, and the constant demand for novelty sex, has all but killed off the happy chickens in the Hong Kong sex market. This competition means customers can now use hookers' bodies at historically low prices. It has become a buyer's market – a man's market, which reinforces the position of the conservative feminist who asserts that prostitution belongs to a patriarchic culture.

While the 'happy chicken' notion is directly opposed to the stereotype of the 'wretched hooker', it overlooks the need for a veil of misery, which often helps prostitutes in their business. During my interviews, the hookers served me 24-flavour bitter tea to ensure I would taste their bile. Money-driven street hookers would say, "I'm a better interview candidate. My story is sadder." The comment that most effectively spoke for the group was, "Everybody is pitiful! The more pitiful you are, the more you can charge."

Interviewees were often disappointed by my lack of reaction to their pitiable plight, by the apparent absence of compassion or mercy. "Isn't that enough material for you to show a real tragedy?" they would ask. It was often only over a beer, after they had used up their prepared lines, that I would reap a surprise harvest of more genuine material.

The heavy make-up of night girls presents a superficial image of enthusiasm, but is nothing more than a means to satisfy men's ideas of availability. The ever-present flirtation and hustle are just part of a mechanical business operation. Hookers cannot say whether this career caters for or hurts them; it is just business. The old saying goes, "You always hate what you do." Hookers also hate their job, but like anyone else, they do it for the money. Prostitutes have their own survival techniques. They know that – just like customers – women's organisations, social workers, charity agencies, church groups, writers and reporters all want to believe that hookers are miserable, not decadent, women. If you have a fat purse, they will agree with your arguments that a donkey is a horse, and if you can sign a big enough cheque, the donkey could well be a monkey.

People generally believe that hookers suffer from social discrimination. Nightclub madams and hostesses tend to say the following:

- Their social circle is made up of their peers.

- Their interactive social relationships are with the customers, who come to buy joy. If they are mean to the hookers, it reduces their own pleasure, so they generally give them face.

- Hong Kong society looks down on poverty, not on prostitutes. The entertainment news is filled with reports on how hotshot stars – TV people, celebrity women and models – strike transparent sex deals.

- If they have made a fortune, they have no fear of disclosing their profession.

- With good money and independence, a star hostess does not have to flatter a boss, and may have frequent contact with powerful tycoons. They have little respect for women clerks, secretaries or accountants.

Top-class hookers usually adopt two methods to avoid social discrimination: first, a vague positioning of themselves, so they can laugh at other hookers to cover up their own prostitution; and second, simple confidence – they avoid behaving like victims.

It's an undeniable fact that hookers are reluctant to reveal their identities. One factor is social discrimination, but there are three other less obvious factors which cannot be ignored. Not every hooker can make big money; if a hooker doesn't make big money, she loses face. Average-looking girls fear comments like "How can you sell yourself, looking like that?" And underground prostitution may protect their privacy.

A volatile emotional life is the root cause of a hooker's sorrows. Emotionally vulnerable hookers often look upon their lovers as the sole purpose of their lives and their sole source of happiness. This makes them particularly vulnerable at the break-up of personal relationships, and easy targets for others who would swindle them out of their money.

They tend to buy expensive love and look for substitutes like drugs and gambling. Consequently, they may eventually end up as deadbeats with drug addictions. When they are happy chickens, they use gigolos to satisfy their emotional needs. When they feel at a low point, they will pay for even more expensive gigolos to try to heal their emotional wounds, only to be battered more badly.

Hong Kong hookers do not need prostitutes' rights, which cannot guarantee the love-hungry hooker a stable companion or otherwise satisfy her need for true love. The prostitution issue involves the whole range of social and cultural attitudes to sex. The marriage system has nurtured an ideology which puts virginity, love, sex and marriage together in one category, and this is exactly the origin of both hookers' business and their emotional problems.

Specialised psychological assistance would be of far more help to Hong Kong prostitutes than a fight for legal protection. Part of the argument for happy whoredom is the assumption that prostitutes' rights would also guarantee customers' wellbeing. My findings, however, indicate that customers would prefer things to remain as they are. This is because openly established rights and decriminalisation would remove the exciting element of naughtiness found in the search and covert enjoyment of commercial sex.

Dear Mr Customer, how you relish prowling around after prostitutes! Enjoy the illicit thrill!

Dear Miss Hooker, fuck on, the burning pit of hell isn't so bad!

# 18

## FROM THE OUTSIDE LOOKING IN

Since conducting the original interviews that provided material for the Chinese version of *Whispers and Moans*, it has been possible to collect experiences and comments from Western expatriates. Their views provide a response to the proposition by Hong Kong prostitutes in an earlier chapter that Western men make up the lowest class of clientele.

The majority of the informants for this chapter work at senior management level or are professionals of various kinds. The strongest impression is of their surprise at the prevalence of prostitution in Hong Kong and other Asian cities. In their home countries, prostitution obviously exists, but it is not ordinarily offered as part of business entertainment.

Western men say that using commercial sex services is typically not something that is readily admitted to. Indeed, the majority of men would have a lower opinion of another man if they were to learn he used prostitutes. Rather than a moral judgement, it would simply be seen as a sign of inadequacy.

John is a 60-year-old British expatriate who has spent almost 20 years in Hong Kong. He divorced his English wife to marry a Hong Kong woman he met overseas. The new couple returned here to start a business. They subsequently divorced. Since that time, he has tried many of the offerings of the Hong Kong sex industry.

"Just beware. First, you think: here is a cute little woman, more feminine and a lot slimmer than you will find in the UK these days. But after a while, you realise the expectations are all different. The emphasis is on the material, and on immediate gain. There seems little interest in taking a longer-term view. Even romantic gestures need a material token as evidence.

"I'm getting on a bit now, and being single, after two divorces, I have decided to avoid long-term involvements. It took some effort to overcome my instinctive reluctance, but after I went to a few nightclubs here, and had a few massages and so on, it's now not a problem. I see in the commercial approach echoes of what I found in my marriage. In the end, you realise that in a culture without organised welfare, individuals can rely only on themselves or on their families. If there is a problem in the family background, people can end up being very calculating and materialistic, simply because it is a matter of personal survival. In a marriage, the man is the welfare system. If he is not career-minded, and earns less than his neighbour, he is seen as less of a man, and the woman loses face.

"Chinese women will go on and on about finding romantic love – but when they have it, they don't know its value, because they can't quantify it or go shopping with it."

Steve is 49 years old. He has lived in Asia since 1990. He applied for an overseas posting after his divorce.

"I find Chinese women physically very attractive, but there is always a catch. It's hardly a scientific survey, but I have probably had a similar number of western and Asian girlfriends. Asian women like the idea of sex, but seem uncomfortable with the actual activity; in particular, they are uncomfortable with their own anatomy. Once, after intercourse, oral sex was refused because of where my cock had just been. On another occasion, after my partner – who enjoyed kissing – had obviously enjoyed receiving oral sex, she asked me to take a drink of water before kissing her again. She said, "I don't want to taste myself." There's something weird going on there.

"Great sex is great sex in any language, and my experience of the extremes of good and bad in the east and west are probably comparable. The difference in Asia is that the experiences have been either very good or very bad, with nothing inbetween. I guess that's why I find Chinese women attractive; it is the unexpected contrasts. They seem to have the idea that in any given circumstance, there is an appropriate way to behave. There are no grey areas. You can have a very demure, shy, quiet woman who shuns displays of affection in public, but when the bedroom door is closed, turns into not a sex kitten but a sex tigress!"

Jim is a 43-year-old, self-employed British expatriate who has lived in Singapore, Malaysia and Hong Kong.

"I once knew a Malay woman who had divorced and had three children. When she was a child, she had been left with a Chinese family while her parents were out at work during the day. This meant she was able to speak several Chinese dialects quite fluently, very unusual for a Malay.

"After her divorce, and without her husband's income, she struggled to get by on the money she earned from her office job. She was tall and slim, and in incredible shape for a mother of three. She found her way into escort work. Being bright, she knew it couldn't last for long because of her age, and she realised she should find a way of organising her own escort business. I knew her during her separation from her husband and then we lost touch. When we met up again she had become an escort. She was very frank about her experiences, and told me a lot of stories about what the clients wanted, the specialities of the girls she worked with, their likes and dislikes and so forth.

"She thought Chinese girls felt they were superior in some way, and always demanded more money than other nationalities for sex.

"She disliked Chinese and Indian clients; Chinese men because of their lack of manners and general attitude, and Indian men because of body odour. Another reason she disliked Chinese men was their small dicks. She had no patience "trying to work with nothing" and found it difficult to take the client seriously when he was poorly endowed. Chinese men also did not tip well.

"She preferred western clients and older Japanese men. She thought westerners talked too much sometimes about their feelings and problems, but unlike Asian men, they would show concern for her feelings and ask her where she wanted to go and what she wanted to do. She thought they were also generally more thoughtful when it came to sex. She felt she was treated more like an equal.

"She liked the older Japanese men because although they could be arrogant, they were polite with it. They were supposedly not very sexually demanding, and they tipped well.

"Although we still found each other attractive, her escort work was too much for me. Her parting shot was: "Be very careful if you have a Chinese girlfriend. All they want is financial security. Leave Chinese women to Chinese men – they deserve each other."

George is a 38-year-old professional representing a European organisation which provides specialised technical consultancy services.

"In business, in Asia, you can be offered a girl after dinner just like you might be offered a coffee in the west. Of course prostitution exists in the west, but you have to go and look for it, for yourself. I was in the construction industry in the UK and Europe for about 20 years and never once came across prostitution. Maybe you would be invited to a golf club, or to go sailing, that was it. In Hong Kong, it is a way of life, even among younger men who you might think would be more educated.

"Once, I was in a group sitting around a table after dinner. There were eight of us, including a local businesswoman. I was embarrassed for her because the local men started talking about women and prostitutes without any compunction. She later told me it was quite normal, and she regularly shrugged it off. She also explained it was why she had a western boyfriend, and would never look at another Chinese man.

"The men were discussing where they would go to find women when they left the restaurant. One of the men who had spent time in the West looked at me and said, for all to hear, "George may not want to, he's western." I think it was meant to imply I was a sissy of some kind. There were comments such as "It's no big thing, I'm happily married but it doesn't stop me. If I find a girl, it's just entertainment, it's all over and forgotten by tomorrow morning. I go home, my wife doesn't know. Everything is OK."

"Anyway, one of the local men, who had too much beer, and regularly travelled in mainland China, was starting to boast that he had girlfriends in seven cities. He regularly visited them, and they all waited for his visits and loved him dearly. Then he took out his diary and began to read out their contact details, as evidence he wasn't bullshitting. This was too much for me. I said, "Have you thought, each of those girls might have their own diary, with details of seven boyfriends?" He realised what I was saying and emphatically told me, without any trace of irony, "Of course they don't! They all love me!"

David is a furniture designer in his sixties who has lived and worked in Asia for many years.

"It was a shock, when I first started to visit Asian cities, to be the subject of frequent soliciting, which I had never experienced in Europe. Even so, one event will stay in my memory as an extreme example of the art of marketing!

"I needed to discuss some business with a friend. I was based in Hong Kong, and he was travelling through the region, but not to Hong Kong. The compromise was to meet for a day in Singapore. We stayed in a hotel on Orchard Road – the city's main shopping street. After dinner, we decided to take a stroll along the road and back to the hotel. It was around 11:00pm, the street was well lit, and like many Asian cities, was still very alive at that time of night.

"One end of the road was quite leafy. As the two of us walked by, we heard: "Psst!" Looking around, we saw nothing, and continued. After another couple of steps, there was a more insistent "Psst!" This time, when we turned around, there was a skimpily dressed girl standing in the greenery. As we looked at her, she smiled, and pulled up her top to show us her breasts. We sighed, turned around, and continued walking. Then there was a frantic "Psst. Psst. Psssssst!" When we looked a second time, she had pulled up her short skirt to reveal herself in her full, pantiless glory."

Kevin, 40, sells specialised chemical products manufactured by a German company.

"I had been a self-employed consultant in the UK. I later worked for a company that sent me to Asia. One of my previous clients from my self-employed days had retired and was doing a world tour, and was passing through Hong Kong. He and his wife, and my girlfriend and I, went for dinner not far from his hotel. After dinner, we were walking back to his hotel as a foursome.

"Nearby, there was a group of young girls, probably about 12 to 14 years old. They had been watching us as he and I paused to stand still and chat, falling a few yards behind the women. It was then the girls approached us, and said, "You like young girls? You like to know us better? We come back to your hotel?"

"I didn't know whether I was more shocked by the girls' age, or by the fact they had knowingly approached us virtually within earshot of my friend's wife and my girlfriend."

Maurice is a 35-year-old engineer who started visiting Hong Kong in his mid-twenties.

"I had never been offered girls as business entertainment before coming to Hong Kong. But here, it was just like going for a beer after work. I had heard stories of loss of business when surprised westerners had openly rejected the offer of women, saying they were happily married and had no interest in girls, which caused a public loss of face for the host.

"This is why now I will never accept an offer of dinner from a business contact, to avoid this type of situation. Lunch is OK, but not dinner.

"The first time, I was completely green. I was a junior member of staff of a UK company sent to help a senior manager present an exhibition in association with the company's Hong Kong agent. One evening, my senior colleague and I were taken to what I later learned was a premier nightclub in Hong Kong. I expected a drink, maybe some cabaret, and then go back to my hotel. No sooner had we sat down than girls came and sat beside us all. I was tongue-tied and felt very awkward. I thought if I ignored 'my' girl she would get the message and go away, but she stayed. I tried going to the toilet for a very long time, hoping she would be gone when I returned to the table. That didn't work either. Then I complained of feeling unwell and went out onto a balcony for air. It was then the host came after me, to find out what was wrong and why I didn't like 'my' girl. The best excuse I could think of was that she couldn't speak English very well.

"The host persuaded me to return to my seat, when almost instantly a new girl came to sit by me. Her English was perfect.

"I had some idea about 'loss of face' so I suggested I leave the club with the girl, on our own. The host smiled, pleased that his guest was happy. At the time, I did not realise the host must have paid a buy-out fee for the girl. My hotel was nearby so we walked back.

"She appeared to be a sweet girl, and told me she had to work long hours in the club until after midnight, and then had to wake up at four in the morning to help her aged mother make noodles to sell from the little family noodle stall. The story sounded a bit too pat, which made it easier for me to do what I had already planned.

"When we got back to the hotel, I called over a taxi and put the girl inside. She must have thought we were going on somewhere else. I made it seem like I was about to get into the taxi as well. I gave the driver some money to take the girl home, shut the cab door, and quickly disappeared into the hotel.

"The second time, I didn't see it coming at all. I was invited to an early dinner by a very well educated, respectable client. Previously, my girlfriend and I had been to dinner with him and his wife, along with his British supplier and his wife.

"This time, at a five-star hotel, the early dinner was for just the three of us: my client, the British supplier, and me. After dinner, around 8:30pm, I was saying my goodbyes when my client suggested we have a quick after-dinner drink. Just as we turned the corner to enter the lobby bar, my client stepped forward, towards three seated, really attractive young girls. "Oh, look," he said, "my young friends are here, let's join them."

"I used the 'leave early' ploy, and since then, I have never accepted dinner from a business contact."

Graham is a 37-year-old design consultant, posted to Hong Kong by his UK employer.

"Clients from my UK head office were visiting a local Chinese client of mine. I later learned that the Chinese client took the visitors to a cheesy nightclub, and called girls over to the table. The guys from the UK, unused to this, refused the girls as politely as they could. The local then tried to find out which girls they would find attractive, and asked for several to parade in front of their table. By this time, the guys from the UK told me they felt pretty uncomfortable, and they made their excuses and left.

"The next day, the local client came to my office and vented his anger at me! He was shouting, which is unusual for a Chinese man in business. He complained, very rudely, that my UK clients had caused him to lose face, and what was I going to do about it!"

Geoff is a large, bluff Australian in his sixties. He was divorced 18 years ago and since then has moved around the Asia-Pacific region working on civil engineering projects.

"Here I am, not much to look at and getting on a bit. Life is short and I've got no real roots or family. I never had much success with women when I was younger, so in the last few years I've decided to make the most of things while I've still got my health.

"I've tried girls everywhere I've been. These days I wouldn't give you two cents for a Chinese tart. Either they try to play the innocent girlish type, or they try to play on your sympathy, or they are very matter-of-fact and make no effort at all. The sex is crap. They either lie there like a wet lettuce leaf or they scream and thrash about – making out they've never had it so good. The acting is so bad I don't know whether I should be more embarrassed for myself or for them. In any case, they can't wait to get the sex over with – but maybe that's because of me [laughs].

"Chinese women don't seem to understand that half the world's population has got pussy, and theirs is not the only one on offer. They think they are sitting on Fort Knox.

"With Chinese women, it's like they are not really connected to their pussy. That may be why their personal hygiene can be a bit dodgy. Anyway, there are two of us there, it's taking time out of both our lives, and I make the effort to make sure she's comfortable, but it still reminds me of that scene in the film *Klute*, where Jane Fonda is playing a tart. She looks over the guy's shoulder at her watch while telling him he's screwing like a good 'un.

"Thai girls can be more fun, and so can Filipino girls. They seem to get more fully involved.

"Chinese girls can look good, very slim. If you like the play-acting and the Lolita thing, or the stone-hearted bitch act, or the "I'm a poor thing, pay me more because of my sick mother" story, or the "you are so lucky my pants are off" attitude, then go for it."

Cliff is in his late fifties and owns a large manufacturing company in the British Midlands.

"I only ever went to Asia once. I was staying in a very nice hotel in Hong Kong and there was a pedestrian walkway from the hotel to a shopping mall. It was one of the few days I had time to spare. It was about midday and I thought I would go shopping for something for the family. You have to remember this is a very up-market environment, middle of the day, in broad daylight with other people passing by.

"On the walkway I notice a pretty young woman, who starts to approach me. Innocently I guess she wants the time or something, so I am thrown when she sweetly says, "I come to your hotel room and give you massage?"

"The penny drops: I am being solicited. I don't want to cause a fuss so I quietly refuse and try to walk on. Then she grabs onto me and says, "If you don't say yes, I scream and say you attack me." Now I am worried, but I think as there are people walking by, there will be a witness to back me up. I pull my arm free and walk on. Now she says, "If I come to your room I give you the best blow job of your life!" Now I am desperate to shake her off, so I turn around and say back to her, "I am not interested, because I'm gay, I prefer boys!"

"Without batting an eyelid she calmly says, "I have dick, can also do that."

# 19

## SEX WORKERS, WATCH YOUR STEP

How many prostitutes are there in Hong Kong? Which age group constitutes the majority? For how many years do they normally stay in the profession?

There is no reliably accurate data. Prostitutes are an illegal, transient population, for which no official agency is able to produce precise numbers. If readers need data, they may check with the Hong Kong Police Force, where the anti-vice squad keeps records of arrested prostitutes. It is likely, though, that the number of arrested prostitutes bears little relation to the actual number working.

I have studied sex workers over several years, only to find there is no such thing as a 'prostitute mentality'. The prostitute's world is a microcosm of a gigantic, complicated capitalist society. Maybe I have learned nothing more than if I had written about human psychology under a capitalist system.

Hong Kong sex workers effectively operate underground, initiating business at any time, bargaining anywhere, with strategies to avoid police anti-vice campaigns. There is a mutually supportive, pragmatic sisterhood stronger than the political idealism of any feminist group. The aggregated anger and stress in sex work has developed its own channels. What chickens cannot absorb is taken out on ducks, who then pass it down to cheap street hookers, who ultimately turn to heroin and only consider help from Blue Bird or Purple Vine as a last resort when in terminal decline.

I have been looking for a defender of Hong Kong sex workers' rights, like the Los Angeles police officer Norma Jean Almodovar. I have found none, but have met teenage prostitutes who openly express their sexual and material lust. This mythical Almodovar figure must be exceptionally beautiful and smart, and must be having so much fun that she has no time to fight against discrimination. If she saw the suffering of street hookers, as I have, she might pause and shed a few tears for them.

I have long been bothered by the prostitution paradox, to which I have been unable to find a simple answer. How is it that such a denigrated activity seems to thrive no matter what? I am certain this book will annoy pro-marriage, pro-family moralists, and will equally irritate advocates of sexual liberation.

It can be argued that some marriages stay together because commercial sex provides an outlet for activities that might otherwise distress or alienate a spouse. Indeed, this is an argument often put forward by sex workers seeking to identify their social contribution.

Anyone taking a moralistic view of sex work is necessarily drawing a line between 'good' and 'bad'. Choosing between potential partners, or dating, is a normal enough human pastime. Should there be a choice between two partners, and one is obviously significantly more wealthy, there may be a few raised eyebrows or cynical comments if the wealthy one wins the suit. This choice is an implicit deal, and is within the law.

If, however, the deal is the result of negotiation and the benefits are quantified, some would say we are standing on the brink of prostitution. If one party undertakes a similar negotiation on a regular basis, the majority would describe this as commercial sex. How then does the moralist draw the line? Is the boundary determined by the explicit quantification of benefits, or the frequency of such arrangements, or the nature of the benefits received for sex? Is there a difference between accepting a handful of dollars, or an all-expenses-paid holiday, or a honeymoon and housing for life?

Whether marriage is simply a single sex-for-benefits deal, or an individual is able to regularly repeat the deal with other consenting adults, the fundamental drive is the same – survival.

Writing *Whispers and Moans* has given me insights into the relationships between prostitutes and sex culture, sex culture and social order, social order and human development, and human development and sex strategies. These interactions have driven much of human social evolution.

It is important to accept that sex workers are a symptom of the workings of a culture, and not a cause of its moral decline. Rather than controlling or legislating against sex workers, effort is probably better spent on sex education and encouraging couples to communicate – in short, taking the smutty mystery and notions of shame out of sex.

I have considered the situation of my informants, who I now presume to call brothers and sisters, and must apologise to them for not being able to help them find a dignified existence. I have learned to admire their honesty about their desires. The route through the world of prostitution is strewn with difficulties and I will try to signpost the pitfalls I have discovered along my own journey.

I worked with Blue Bird to write the pamphlet *Street Prostitution, Not Pretty*. All 5,000 copies were distributed among Hong Kong sex workers free of charge. The leaflet used primary education level Cantonese with cartoon illustrations to talk about the failure or success of four local hookers. At the end of each story, I posed the following topics for discussion:

1) Kam To's Expensive Youth – Please do the sums: How much did she overspend in her six months of extravagance? How many years will it take to pay back the debt?

2) The Price of Ah Ching's Love – Why is the hostess's love so intense? If Ah Ching loved herself a little more, and her man a little less, would she have had a better ending?

3) Ah Ming's Momentary Joy – Why do hostesses crave thrills? If there is no plan for the future, will life always be carefree?

4) Ah Choi's Healthy Prostitution – How can Ah Choi save money while enjoying dignity and her work?

The pamphlet *Street Prostitution, Not Pretty* was a hit among Hong Kong sex workers, who would discuss the stories and remark wistfully:

"I was just like that…"

"I'd have turned out better if I had done that…"

"It would have been different if I hadn't done that…"

"I know what's best for me, but I just can't do it…"

The success of the little book reflected the urgent need for psychological guidance for Hong Kong sex workers.

Did it really take so much effort to produce the simple idea of a need for psychological help? Isn't this intentionally trying to depoliticise prostitution and turn it back into a personal issue? Hey! Shouldn't I at least be able to produce an analysis using some grandiose term like 'patriarchal regime'? What is patriarchy anyway?

Patriarchy is a cultural mindset – a mainstream cultural power forging men and women into stereotyped images. This power is preserved in the institution of marriage, which serves to lock men into the position of breadwinner. Women who look for security in marriage have always been instrumental in the construction of the rules and norms of patriarchy. As a lazy term, 'patriarchy' deflects people's attention from the basic question: Are men repressing women or is it culture that is repressing women? Is it men who have created this culture, and do women also benefit from it? Is it men who like to pass off their negative feelings onto prostitutes, or is it wives labelled as 'good women' who like to stigmatise prostitution to draw attention to their own relative virtue?

The prostitutes I met all wanted to move out of the business to marry or to live a conventional family life. The expensive prostitutes I met often bullied cheap hookers, and would deride their poor cousins' ideas of finding happiness in marriage.

In the same way that individuals may be addicted to danger and excitement, alcohol, food or drugs, there appears to be an element of addictive behaviour among commercial sex workers. Despite complaints about working conditions, northern girls, badly behaved clients, low fees, and police harassment, sex workers stay in the business. It's rather like gambling: the next bet, the next horse, the next customer and I will hit the jackpot. I will never have to worry about money; I can retire, experience romantic love, and enjoy a life of luxurious leisure.

Herein lies the basic flaw. The next customer may be fabulously wealthy, but may also be a serial purchaser of commercial sex and have little endurance for monogamous relationships. He may also purchase sex commercially because he has to – as he is unattractive, has bad breath, has poor hygiene, or is an inept lover.

Norma Jean Almodovar has spelled out a truth: "Being a prostitute is a matter of personal choice." Individuals have been freed from traditional culture, taking care of their own responsibilities, thus facing the risks of making choices in many and varied aspects of daily life.

Can Hong Kong sex workers be saved by a politically motivated liberation campaign? Probably not. As a group, sex workers may appear to support political changes made to benefit them. In a one-on-one interview, an individual may express a more personal agenda.

The advent of 2006 saw another casualty of the general state of the Hong Kong economy and competition in its various forms from mainland China. Club Bboss, once the largest Japanese-style hostess nightclub in the world, closed its doors for the last time. It opened in 1984 and dazzled customers with a floor area of 70,000 square feet, seating for 3,000, and an electrically powered, full-sized replica of an antique Rolls-Royce that delivered customers to their seats.

There were three nightly stage shows between 9:00pm and midnight, presented on a rotating stage to give all the customers a chance to ogle the scantily clad performers. Scores of hostesses were available for the male clientele to chat and flirt with. Big spenders could buy hostesses out from the club for the evening.

Subsequently, several other mega-scale hostess nightclubs opened in Tsim Sha Tsui and Wan Chai, acting as a testament to Hong Kong's economic success during the 1980s and 1990s. In recent years, these nightclubs too have experienced decline, facing similar forms of competition. Hong Kong clubs have struggled to survive, reducing both their size and their operating costs. This scaling down is an indicator of the health of the Hong Kong sex industry. While local clubland becomes increasingly barren, nightspots larger than have ever been seen in Hong Kong are opening in southern China.

With the closure of sumptuous nightclubs, competition from northern girls and local part-time sex workers, and customers who have come to expect supermarket rather than boutique prices, the high-priced prostitute is a dying breed. Making a living out of sex is surely becoming as demanding as any other form of work in Hong Kong, now that its economy is in the shadow of China.

Ladies and gentlemen! Brothers and sisters! Chickens and ducks! Thank you for your interviews. If you are smart and capable enough to cope with the demands of the sex business, and fend off the invasion of northern girls, is there anything that can stop you? If you have the looks and the right mentality, and are ready to prey on society, perhaps you will find that prostitution is indeed a win-win game of sex and money. Nobody will be entitled to look down on you.

Maybe you feel you are not respected in the cold light of day, but don't be afraid, because you hold the mystic chip – sex – with which you can gamble your whole life. Being a winner, or a loser, is in your grasp.

To all you newcomers to the business, I respect your nerve and determination, and I am sure you will laugh at poverty, but remember the three biggest traps: dying for face, dying for love, and living for today without a plan for tomorrow.

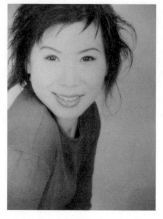 Yeeshan Yang comes from a migratory family background. She spent her childhood years in Maoist China, where she saw her Indonesian-Chinese father politically persecuted as a spy; grew up in Hong Kong; studied Japanese in Tokyo; experienced migrant life again in Australia; then returned to Hong Kong. She has worked in journalism, filmmaking and publishing while conducting anthropological research.

Stories from *Whispers and Moans* have been adapted into two motion pictures: *Whispers and Moans* and *True Women For Sale*, which won Best Actress at the Golden Horse Film Awards.